# 4 Steps to Healthy

## to

## A PARENTING GUIDE

By Heidi J. Moore, MD

Previously titled *F is for Fat, not forever.*

# table *of* contents

# ‑ACKNOWLEDGEMENTS‑

Many people made this guide possible, and I worry that by creating a list of thank-yous, I will leave someone out. But I would be remiss if I didn't publicly acknowledge the following:

- The librarians at Champlain Valley Physicians Hospital, Bonnie and Chris, who must have found all the journal articles ever written about obesity and were able to deliver them to my e-mail inbox quickly, often within a day of my request.

- Karen and Leita, who were at the forefront of ADK 2015 and were on the front lines making change happen in our community.

- David Beguin, a fellow pediatrician who also wanted to change the way our community fought obesity and to change the way we delivered healthcare. He has been at my dining room table more than once, talking about healthcare reform, ADK 2015, and the manuscript itself. There wouldn't be a parenting guide without his friendship.

- Lisa Mecham and Kathryn Rhett, who have impeccable editorial skills.

- Fred Leebron who saw the value in a manual like this.

- My family, who has tolerated hours of my isolation in the "back room" typing away.

- Finally, to my patients. Thank you.

# ~INTRODUCTION~

This was created as a how to guide for parents who wanted to help their children achieve a healthy weight. But the principles involved in helping a child achieve an optimum weight are the same needed for him to have a healthy lifestyle; what started as a weight loss manual for kids is actually a parenting blueprint for raising children who can be healthy. There's still lots in here about how to reverse unhealthy trends, and in fact, I'll start with a story about what motivated me to write this. But the truth is my end goal was never to teach kids how to lose weight; it was to show parents how to raise healthy kids.

I work in upstate New York and have practiced pediatric medicine in the "North Country" for over a decade. My patient mix is almost equally split between privately insured and state insured (Medicaid) and my office is located in Plattsburgh, a medium-sized town at the base of the Adirondack Mountains. It's a beautiful place to live, but the geography and climate bring specific issues that affect the health of my patients. When I first arrived in town, an older doctor crassly introduced me to the weight problem in the local community by telling me that I would need to start using the "North Country unit" of weight measurement, which would be in 200-pound increments.

Not long after, I realized that weight was the factor that would affect my patients' health the most. But it doesn't just affect my patients. Obesity is estimated to cost anywhere from $150 billion[1] to $190 billion[2] a year in the United States, over 20% of total healthcare dollars spent. Every day as a pediatrician, I talked to patients and parents about weight charts and diets

[1] Eric A. Finkelstein, Justin G. Trogdon, Joel W. Cohen, and William Dietz, "Annual Medical Spending Attributable to Obesity: Payer- and Service-Specific Estimates," Health Affairs (Millwood) 28, no. 5 (2009): w822-31.

[2] John Cawley and Chad Meyerhoefer, "The Medical Care Costs of Obesity: An Instrumental Variables Approach," Journal of Health Economics 31, no. 1 (2012): 219-30.

and exercise ad nauseam, but it didn't seem to matter. They kept gaining weight no matter what I said. I tried to be more sympathetic since the task of losing or even maintaining their weight overwhelmed them, and I suspect they dreaded a return visit to my office. They would have to get back on the scale again to review the numbers and justify why they had not lost. Patients cried when we talked about their weight. I told myself that their emotions were a testament to us and the connection we had. They trusted me so much that they would let down their guard and share their frustrations and emotional vulnerability.

**No matter how much I wanted to**,
I couldn't follow my patients home.
I couldn't stand beside their chairs as they
**reached for another scoop** of potatoes
and use my megaphone to ask them,
*"Are you sure you want*
*another helping?"*

But their weight didn't seem to change much no matter how much they cried; if anything, the numbers went up, and besides, who wants to be the doctor who makes patients cry? I wanted to help them live healthier lives, not give them the final nudge off an emotional breakdown cliff.

The problem as I saw it at first was that I couldn't follow my patients home. I couldn't live for them. I couldn't throw my body at the next juice drink and knock it out of their hands like some Heisman Trophy candidate might have done. I couldn't carry a megaphone around when they went back for seconds and thirds of mac and cheese and mashed potatoes.

"REALLY?" I would shout through the orange cone. "WHY DON'T YOU WAIT AND SEE HOW YOU FEEL IN ANOTHER TEN MINUTES?"

I wondered whether my voice would matter anyhow. All the forces of the universe seemed aligned against the patients I cared about. For one thing, we live in the part of the country that has six months of winter. Exercise between November and May involves shivering. We huddle over steaming mugs of hot chocolate to keep our energy up, and we entertain ourselves with the next reality show starring someone whose name rhymes with Rookie. And while we watch TV, we console our chilly souls with Michigan sauce and Fluffernutter sandwiches.

So even if I could follow the kids home and body-slam soda and hot dogs and any bread baked without whole grain, eventually I would have to go home to my own children, and eventually my patients would succumb to real life. Again. Their parents were just as disheartened. It wasn't as if they didn't know the information I was spouting at them.

One parent held up her hand like a stop sign and said, "I know, I know. More fruits and veggies, less TV, more exercise."

Knowledge for the most part wasn't the deficit. I could list a million facts about nutrition, and on some level, maybe not the biochemical or cellular physiology level, but on the macro level, the big picture, the majority of parents knew what their kids needed to be healthy. I wasn't bringing anything new to the table.

> **Most parents knew** *what their kids needed to be healthy.* **I didn't need to lecture them** *about facts.*

About the same time that I was feeling the worst about my ability to help my patients, the physicians in my community entered into a groundbreaking pilot of healthcare reform, the Adirondack Region Medical Home

Pilot[3]. It was an agreement between insurance companies, both private and public (Medicare and Medicaid were included), and practicing physicians. If the doctors focused on managing patients who had certain chronic diseases while also focusing on preventive care, and if the offices all became certified as medical homes through NCQA[4], the insurance companies would reimburse us at a higher rate. Since physicians in our community were significantly underpaid compared with the rest of the country, and since we had just experienced a hemorrhage of providers leaving the region, increasing reimbursement sounded like a dream.

## WHERE'S YOUR MEDICAL HOME?

**A medical home isn't a place. It's a philosophy and a way to deliver healthcare that puts the patient's needs first while maintaining the highest level of clinical standards possible.**

The money would allow us to utilize more resources for our patients with chronic illnesses, and it would allow us to recruit more physicians. The pilot began in 2010 and was set to end in 2015. A colleague and I advocated for childhood obesity to be one of the six chronic diseases for our community to focus on.

A small group of doctors, nurses, social workers, County Health Department representatives, and administrators from the medical home pilot began to meet every other week. We brainstormed about the disease process of obesity. If we were going to fix the problem in our community, what would it take?

The Health Department representative came up with a Logic model. It was... well, logical. The social worker talked about all the barriers to

[3] Adkmedicalhome.org

[4] National Committee for Quality Assurance is a nonprofit organization dedicated to improving the quality of healthcare.

care that children and families faced. That was helpful, but depressing. The pediatricians talked about how what the families needed was a coach, a trainer, an advocate, some type of a shaman who would minister to the families as they made habit changes.

In the end, we left the meetings feeling connected to each other, but not very empowered, and the families didn't feel anything. The truth is we were just beginning to explore the complexity of the obesity problem. In our offices, we still spouted information to our patients about why they should change, but to throw salt in the wound, we decided that perhaps we should order blood tests to screen for diabetes and elevated cholesterol. The kids might not lose weight, by golly, but they were going to get stuck with needles on a regular basis. Not exactly incentive to change in the first few months.

| A | Activity |
|---|---|
| D | Dietary choices |
| K | Keeping a balance |
| 2 | Screen time/breast-feeding |
| 0 | Sugar-sweetened beverages |
| 1 | Activity |
| 5 | Fruits and vegetables |

We looked at other models for change, lots of other models. In fact, as we looked around, it seemed that the whole country was approaching the problem piecemeal and each community was coming up with its own micro study to add to the knowledge base of what would or wouldn't work. The encouragement from colleagues was abysmal. I attended one memorable conference in which the speaker said, tongue in cheek, that if anyone wants to give up on saving money in healthcare, they should focus on pediatric issues, and if they're going to waste their time doing that, they might as well focus on childhood obesity. Since that lecture, I've gotten to know the speaker, and I like him a lot. But with his dry sense of humor that day, he highlighted the futility I felt about trying to change obesity. *Kill me now,* I thought. *I'm the captain of a sinking ship.* Because if my community was going to do anything other than enter the beluga whale look-alike contest or race each other to see who gets to the diabetes finish line first, we were going to have to fix the obesity problem, no matter whether it saved us money in the short term or not.

Don't get me wrong. I have very little moral high ground to stand on. Follow me around for a day and you'll understand all my weak points surrounding a healthy lifestyle. Plus, I don't want to be the pediatrician who pretends she's the perfect mother or perfect nutritionist or perfect anything, and I'm fine admitting that not long ago I ate a bag of leftover red and green holiday jelly beans for breakfast while I drove to a community obesity meeting. It was July. I'm also a failed vegetarian. Twice over. I want to be a vegetarian, but not quite as much as I want a really juicy steak.

Still, I didn't feel like I was the most unlikely doctor to lead the charge against childhood obesity. I do lots of things right, even though I do some other things really badly. What I could give to my patients was not the example of perfection, but rather the voice of moderation, reason, and practicality. Maybe, I thought, by admitting all my weak points (or at least some of them) I would gain some validity. Maybe by telling people that I hide candy corns on the top shelf of the pantry where my kids can't find them, or by admitting that for the past two years I've pretended that every vegetable was an airplane or a tiger or a bunny rabbit so my kids would eat them, people would sit up and listen and say, "Oh. I guess she knows."

*"The problem of obesity is complex, but* **the solution is simple."** }

What really drove me crazy when our community considered ways to change the obesity trend was that I did know, and my colleagues knew, that very simple principles led to weight loss in overweight children. Despite the myriad forces against weight loss, success depended on just a few things, the same things identified by other pilots, the same things that parents knew in their hearts as truths of healthy living. So one day, while out mowing the grass, I considered the numbers. I thought about our pilot. And I decided we didn't have anything to lose. A paper bag blew by, and I grabbed it. I scribbled down the abbreviation for the Adirondacks, ADK, and the year the pilot was scheduled to end, 2015. It would be a starting point for us. Something to hang our hats on, so to speak. Something for the community to promote, a single point of reference for us to work toward with patients. A rallying cry to fight against obesity.

{ Parents have *everything they need* to help their children get to a *healthy weight*.

With every patient who came into my office after that, either with or without a weight problem, I began to discuss the four simple concepts of healthy living, the activities represented by ADK 2015. I asked patients to pick one number or one letter to work on and I tried to focus my interviews and education on what I perceived as the family's readiness to change. I attended conferences on motivational interviewing, and I stopped spewing facts. Instead, I began to listen to what my patients had to say.

They had known what to do all along. They had most of the knowledge required to change. Now though they needed motivation and resources to make it happen. After a few more months of listening to my patients, I had another epiphany. They usually didn't even need the resources. They already had them. Maybe they didn't think they did, but with a little more self-discovery they'd be okay. They would realize that they had everything they needed to help their children lead healthy lives. But in the moment they felt overwhelmed with the enormity of the problem and couldn't see their way to make small steps that would pay off in big results. The only thing that was truly lacking was motivation.

And then something that felt like a miracle happened. The first patient I knew of during a decade of practicing medicine walked into my office for a weight check, and she had lost weight!!! Okay, maybe I'd had patients before who had lost weight, but they were infants, and I'd had to admit them to the hospital to check for genetic disorders. At the risk of sounding like the worst doctor on the face of the earth, I will say that in 10 years, if I had an overweight patient who lost weight, the memory of her has been squashed by all the patients who didn't lose. Finally, I had a success story. I weighed her twice on check-in, and then a third time as she walked out the door.

She was incredulous that I would doubt the numbers. "We talked about what to do," she said.

"I didn't think you'd actually do it," I said.

She laughed. "Well, it worked."

After her, more patients who had lost weight came into my office, but more important than changing their numbers, they reported healthier lifestyles.

A year into the pilot, not all my overweight patients had changed, not even the majority, but enough had altered their lifestyles for me to realize that what the patients had been missing all this time was someone to encourage them and motivate them to change. The combination of readiness to change and the micro steps of implementing small lifestyle changes over time had turned the tide for my patients.

Finally, I knew what was missing for the rest. Although a few parents still wanted a quick fix for their children's lives, most were tired of the next greatest thing or the newest fad or the next supplement that promised impossible results and achieved nothing. My patients could see me every three months for weigh-ins, accountability checks, and encouragement, but they needed something on a daily basis to help keep them focused. And while there were plenty of manuals out there about nutrition, most focused on individual aspects of nutrition or the latest flash-in-the-pan fad that wouldn't give any long-term benefit to anyone. What patients needed was a take-home guide for healthy living and encouragement. A manual and a resource to thumb through daily and help focus their efforts, to help them keep their eyes on the long-term goal of healthy living. They were smart enough and engaged enough to commit to do the hard work.

# { *"Fat"is an Ugly Word.*

This book is the manual that will help patients with individual goals, but also with the larger goal of a healthy lifestyle. There's a myriad of factors to consider surrounding pediatric obesity. In fact, whole books are written about tiny aspects of weight management and healthy living, and it's possible to dive into any one area and spend a few eons. But since I'd rather spend time getting my eyebrows waxed as opposed to talking about red dye or yellow dye or, God save me, Vitamin D, we're going to talk about the big picture. We'll dive into four general areas for a while (someone's going to have to pull me up when I start talking about the color spectrum and how it relates to a healthy diet – I love that stuff!), but we won't spend too much time in the weeds. Ultimately, this book isn't about calories, or fiber, or gluten or trans-fatty fats. This is about balance. It's about taking a trip to the Island of Healthy Living and making sure the trip isn't just a vacation.

As I was considering the possibilities of writing a parenting guide, I saw another patient. She was similar to the others, and so overweight at age 9 that she couldn't climb onto the exam table without assistance. We talked about weight charts and goals, and even though she cried a little when she talked about how mean people were to her, I felt encouraged since she and her family seemed ready to take small steps toward the larger goal of health. But when I closed the exam room door and stood on the other side charting, I overheard their conversation.

"You know what the doctor just said, don't you?" the girl's father said. "She said you're fat."

I put my head down on the table outside. I didn't say she was fat. I would never say that. I care too much about my patients to use such an ugly word with them. But others use that word, even others who love them. This parenting guide will help you find your own motivation for change and help as you keep your eyes (and your child's eyes) both focused on the goals you set. It will give step-by-step directions for taking a child or teenager from an unhealthy red zone BMI of > 99% and bringing him or her down into the green zone. Just as importantly, it will give all parents the four steps to keep their children healthy.

And on a personal level, for that girl who has no idea I heard what her father said, it will give her a comeback. And the next time someone calls her fat, she can say, "But it's not forever." Healthy, however, can be.

# ～PART I～

# Our Destination –
# The Island Of
# Healthy Living

# ~CHAPTER 1~

# Get Your Ticket – We're Going On A Trip!

The next part of the book is about how to effect specific change. How to take four concepts that are simple in theory and apply them to the complexity of life. The experience will be a lot like taking a trip.

Let's say you want to travel around the world. Every trip starts with just a few steps, and that's what you're doing now by opening this parenting guide. You want your family to go on a trip, and your destination is the Island of Healthy Living. The island has a very pleasant breeze, mountains set back from a beautiful shoreline, and peaceful rolling ocean waves that only swell to significant size if you want to use a surfboard.

Healthy Living has lots more, though. It has little tiki bars that serve up self-esteem and satisfaction, and a tasty drink called happiness. Sounds idyllic, right? "Heck yeah!" you say. "Get me some tickets!"

I agree, the island is awfully nice, but now I have to tell you the part you probably already knew – after all, you've watched enough kitchen gadget commercials to know that something that good comes with a price. The price for the ticket to the Island of Healthy Living is change.

"Ugh," you say. Maybe you aren't entirely happy with where you live now, but at least you're familiar with it. You've gotten used to the traffic noises from the interstate you live under and the subway you live on top of. When you consider everything involved in the move, you might argue that you really don't mind the early morning supersonic jet noises from the local airport, and you're even fond of your neighbor who is always yelling at his pet python because it ate the cat, again. Actually, with change as the price of the ticket, you aren't at all sure that you want to move.

## WHEN TO CALL IN THE EXPERTS

This book was written to help you make the trip to the island, to help you change, to fill a void that existed, a gap between the doctor's office (my office specifically) and your home. But I need to back up for a second and caution that sometimes you'll need more than a parenting guide. Most of the time, you'll apply specific steps here, and you'll wake up in a year with the happy problem of having to buy new clothes at your island home. Your family's waistlines will be shrinking, and they will have worn out the last three pairs of hiking boots and will need more. But sometimes this book won't be enough. Specifically, you may need extra help in the areas of sensory disorders[9], exercise risk, and mental health.

For instance, when you get to Chapter Five and the number 5, if your child can't adjust to a variety of textures or tastes no matter how patient you are and no matter how slowly you introduce change, it may be worth considering medical problems and sensory disorders as a source of the difficulty. Your child may be trying to eat broccoli but can't physically swallow anything lumpy. If you're making the necessary changes in your family's lifestyle and not seeing results, it's worth getting an outside (objective) opinion on why you might be up against a wall.

If your child has both obesity and significant learning disabilities, someone needs to evaluate him for specific genetic syndromes such as Prader-Willi[10], and just as with adults, there's an important cardiac risk evaluation that needs to take place before a really out-of-shape child begins an exercise program. When you start to work on Chapter Four and the number 1, it's not going to be enough for an overweight child to wander into the gym and have someone chase behind him yelling to run faster. That's one reason why weight-loss programs based on medical and scientific evidence regarding exercise and nutrition are the best of all worlds.[11] They are safer. They also are exceedingly rare for children.

---

[9] Sensory disorders are likely to be a symptom of other issues, and the diagnosis of sensory-processing disorders is complex and not yet agreed upon. Pediatrics 129, no. 6 (2012): 1186-89.

[10] Pediatrics 91, no. 2 (1993).

[11] Kids Underground is one program that I've seen like that. It's a family-based model with safety checkpoints built in so someone who has as much fat content in his cardiac muscle as in his derriere is less likely to keel over from a coronary when he starts a kickball game.

> **PRADER-WILLI SYNDROME** is associated with
> rapid weight gain and obesity as a toddler, mild to moderate
> mental retardation or learning problems in older children,
> and hypogonadism (small genitalia). Children affected by this
> syndrome consume large amounts of food and are obsessed with it,
> even stealing or hoarding it.
>
> Specific criteria for the disorder include "major" and "minor"
> characteristics.

The issue of needing outside help is never more apparent than when there are mental health issues associated with obesity. I have very few obese patients who are completely free of mood disorders, but depression and anxiety is usually secondary to the obesity, and those problems resolve themselves when the child reaches a healthier weight. However, if the depression or anxiety are the primary problems and the obesity is secondary, we could talk about the four aspects of a healthy lifestyle until we're blue, and your child won't be able to make any changes.

{ **"Pre-participation" exams:** *exams done before someone starts an exercise program or joins a sports team, should assess blood pressure, flexibility, and strength.*

In my office, we can refer patients to a mental health counselor who is part of our office work flow, and although sometimes I have trouble getting patients to agree to go ("What do you think – that I'm fat and crazy?"), the ones who do go benefit immensely. If we were able to remove the stigma of mental illness from patients, obesity would decrease as well, because families would feel free to get help in all aspects required to have a healthy lifestyle.

# PICKING A PLACE TO START:
## FIND A NUMBER

The next four chapters can stand on their own, as mileposts to the Island of Healthy Living, and there's no compelling reason to start with one specific area. You shouldn't feel like you have to start at the first chapter and move ahead sequentially. It's okay to start at 0 and move on to 5 before you come back to 2. The sections are relatively independent of each other and can be worked through in any order. That said, where to start can be a tough decision.

| 2 | **Screen time** (computer, television, hand-held devices) |
|---|---|
| 0 | **Sugar-sweetened beverages** |
| 1 | **Physical activity** |
| 5 | **Fruits and vegetables** |

There are two points of view, similar to the two ideas parents have about giving their child a flu shot when he's sick. One camp of parents says, "I don't want to give Johnny the flu shot. Poor thing, he already has a cold." The other camp says, "Go ahead and give it. He's sick already. What's a little more misery?" You may want to start your lifestyle changes with an area that's the least painful, one in which your family isn't feeling that bad to start with. For instance, if the only change you need to make in the two-hour screen time section is to take texting away at the dinner table, well, that might be an easy place to start and ensure an emotional rush of accomplishment. On the other hand, you may recognize that for you, the biggest impact and change you can make in your child's lifestyle is to increase fruits and veggies, and even though that will be the most difficult change to make, you want to get the hardest over with first.

Neither approach is wrong. With the former, the risk is that the change will be so incremental that there will be few discernible results, while the risk of the latter approach is that your family may get discouraged and quit before the first two weeks is up.

{ *No matter where you start,*
*begin with a short-term goal in mind.*

No matter where you start, begin slowly with a short-term goal in mind (see Chapter Seven for more about goal setting) and give at least a full two to six weeks of behavior change for small goals and three months for the intermediate-length goals. Also, keep in mind the consequences of "giving in." Let's skip examples about diet and exercise right now and go back to the days of trying to get your child to sleep for more than two hours a clip in the night.

Let's say that in a moment of self-preservation, you decide to let your child "cry it out" to teach him to go to sleep. I'm not talking about pros and cons of this training method, I'm just pointing out behavior responses and what you could expect your child to do based on your own behavior. Let's say you let your 9-month-old cry himself to sleep for two days, but on the third day his cries are breaking your heart. He screams louder and longer than the first two days combined, and you are absolutely certain he'll be in therapy one day talking about why you ruined his life that night in August when he was crying and you wouldn't come get him out of the crib.

Let's say that because of his cries and your fears, on the fateful third day of sleep training you scurry to the bedroom after he cries for 20 minutes and you pick him up. You probably say things like "I'm so sorry. I'll never do that again. You're okay – I've got you." He's finally quiet and falls asleep on your shoulder while making little shuddering sobbing noises as he drifts off, each whimper like a dagger in your resolution.

The next week, he awakens 10 times a night, and if little Bubba Jr. doesn't sleep for longer stretches of time, you're never going to sleep much either, and because of sleep deprivation, you think you'll probably die before he gets out of high school. For his own good, you decide to go back to the sleep training.

You think you'll start back at day four of sleep training, just picking up where you left off, but when you go to put him down alone again, you realize your folly. Now, instead of 20 minutes of crying, he cries for 40 minutes or an hour, and you realize that you're not on day four, you're at day negative five.

By picking him up on the third night, after you "made" him cry himself to sleep on day one and two, you gave an *unpredictable variable response*. Essentially, you did the worst thing you could have done to effect behavior change. You reinforced the behavior that you wanted to get rid of – you cuddled with little Bubba to get him to stop screaming like a banshee, but you did it in an unpredictable way. He didn't know the third day was when you were going to break. But now he knows it's worth crying for an extended time because you're coming to get him eventually.

> *Consistent responses are the keys to **changing your child's behavior.***

To take the example even further, the next worst thing you can do is to resolve again to go back to sleep training, but on the sixth day, after Bubba cries for 50 minutes (which of course feels like five hours), you pick him up and put him to sleep with rocking again. Then he will discover that you may not come on the third day after 20 minutes of crying, maybe it will take five days, maybe 10, but eventually, you're going to break. Unintentionally, you've trained him to cry longer.

Apply the concept of intermittent rewards back to nutrition, although you could just as easily pick screen time or exercise. Let's say you decide that for the next two weeks, your kids are going to use a portion plate, and no matter what, come heck or high water, the meals are getting served in the little slots that give you flashbacks to 1980s cafeteria-style restaurants. The portion plates prove to be a miserable experience for the first two days, although everyone is sort of game. You've done the hard work of getting buy-in and setting goals together (Chapter Seven). But on the third day, there's a dining room table revolt. The kids say you don't love them, and as a matter of fact, they say you actually hate them because they're starving to death, and you don't care that they're withering away in front of you. For your own part, you have no doubts that you must be starving them, because prior to the last few days, they had been eating four to five times the portion sizes you've been spooning out, and half the plate is now taken up with those stupid vegetables that they don't eat anyhow, so really they're down to almost no consumable calories on their plate, and because of you they'll never be happy again, and maybe they will starve to death. At the least – you guessed it – they're going to be in therapy talking about how you ruined their lives.

If at that point you take the portion plates to the front door and use them like you're a contestant in the Frisbee Olympics, well, even if you repent immediately, climb the big pine on the corner of the lot, retrieve the Frisbee portion plates, and tell yourself that tomorrow you'll stick it out no matter what – too bad for you. Because the screaming/crying/pushback factor will be a million times more extreme at the next meal. The kids know that at some point you're going to break and the portion plates are going to become projectiles. Just as in sleep training or any behavior modification, parents should know that every time they "break" and give in, the next time they try to make change stick will be exponentially more difficult. Don't make a change for three days and then renege.

**Find a cheerleader** *to encourage you, and help you stick with your goals! Maybe, by the way, that cheerleader will be online instead of in your house.*

I have one child at home who has the willpower and persistence of a badger. On my frustrated parenting days, I call her stubborn and I refuse to accept responsibility for any genetic tendencies. On my positive days, when I've gotten plenty of rest and have my long-term parenting goals fully in view, I simply say she has strong willpower, a chip off the old block really, and she'll be able to accomplish anything she wants once she learns to focus her energy. Anyhow, on one of my daughter's "badger" days recently, which happened to coincide with one of my poor parenting days, I ended up climbing into my pickup truck, which was parked in the garage. I curled up on the floorboard with my forehead on the passenger seat. The badger wanted a popsicle, which I had already told her she couldn't have, and if I didn't stay out of her line of sight, she was going to wear me down like water on a boulder. So there I was, a professional in child development and behavior, curled up on a floor mat, flattened down so my 3-year-old couldn't find me. It wasn't one of my more stellar moments, but I think it gets the point across: as parents, we have to do what it takes to stand our ground even if it means retreating for a bit. I regrouped, came out of the truck, and was able to out-stubborn her.

**THE NEXT FOUR CHAPTERS** will make schedules based on your personal goals.

**PLAN:** Look at what you're doing now.

**DO:** Make a change for the better.

**CHECK:** Look again to see how you're measuring up to the original plan.

**ACT:** Make changes again, and start all over!

All you need are some index cards and a marker. A timer will help as well. For every section, you'll write down your current numbers, your long-term goal and your medium range goals, and you'll post the index card somewhere that is visible to everyone in the family!

*These schedules will be based on the Deming Model. The idea is that goal setting and behavior changes are not static, but very fluid and need frequent evaluation and tweaking.*

With that in mind, look ahead to see what section you're going to work through first. Which area will be the most difficult for you to hold steady on? Do you know you're going to crumble if the kids beg for another dinner roll? Do you think that after two days of putting vegetables on the plate you'll break down and fill every part of the portion plate with mac and cheese? If so, perhaps you should build success in another area first and come back to the tough areas.

There's no wrong way to do this. If it takes us curling up on a truck floorboard to stay strong and get our families healthy, it's okay.

# ~CHAPTER 2~

# ADK 2015: Shhhh... I Can Hear The Calories Burning

When you begin to make the changes suggested in this chapter, your world will get a whole lot quieter. Imagine the difference between the noise of city traffic and the sounds of... oh, say, an isolated island. On the surface, most people think that decreasing screen time is easy, because we don't have to watch TV right? We can turn it off anytime. Sure. Just like we can stop drinking or smoking anytime we blasted well please thank you very much, just go ahead and change the subject RIGHT NOW.

Chronic television viewing releases brain chemicals comparable to the ones released during chronic overeating, so when we watch too much TV, we feel the way we do when we chronically overeat. The screen-time habit is addictive, and even though we don't necessarily feel good when we keep the TV on for six hours a day, we still do it. We slump into the couch cushions and reach for the remote and begin the thumb-clicking, channel-surfing twitch that is as unfulfilling as the shows we watch when there's "nothing on."

## THE RISK OF DECREASING TV TIME...
### Your kids are going to want something else to do!!!

Think about when you let your kids watch TV . . . likely it's when you really need to get something done: the bills paid, the house cleaned, the conference call for work. TV is a pretty nice way to entertain your kids while you get some other adult stuff out of the way. So when screen time goes down, so does the amount of time you have to do your stuff.

## GOAL: TWO HOURS OR LESS OF SCREEN TIME EVERY DAY

I am not saying that TV is the great evil. I happen to avoid it like the plague since I blink and an hour passes, then I blink again and it's two hours past my bedtime. It may sound like I am trying to convince you otherwise, but some TV is worthy of being designated art. It can be educational. It can be entertaining. But too much TV is a mind-numbing drain on our intelligence and, in my opinion, is largely responsible for the downfall of communication and thoughtful conversations in our families.

| GOAL: What is your screen-time goal? |
|---|
| No TV while eating . . . |
| Only G-rated movie nights . . . |
| No TV on weeknights . . . |

My sister and I have a vivid memory of a summer growing up in Georgia when, by some cable fluke, we got pay TV without actually paying for it. We were almost teenagers and were home alone while our mother worked. Left to our own devices, we watched at least eight hours of television a day, the same movies over and over, sometimes the same one three times in a row. Even now, the theme song to The Pirates of Penzance induces a drugged, unproductive, and sluggish feeling. If I wasn't watching Pirates, I was blasting pixelated space invaders with a joystick on the Atari. My screen time that summer was only interrupted by sleep.

If I consider that summer and compare screen time opportunities then to all the technologies available currently, it's clearly a bigger challenge now to limit screen time. As I write this chapter, I'm listening to my iPod (which has videos if I want to watch them), I have my iPhone out to check text messages, and I have another window open on my computer to check e-mails. Finally, in case a battery dies or a bolt of lightning strikes the other devices, I have my iPad. Apparently, except for the fact that I'm typing on a PC, I'm Apple's fantasy woman. And like all the patients who bring their electronics into the exam room, I'm addicted to the devices.

When we work on the number 2 part of a healthy lifestyle, we have to turn off the TV. The computer. The smartphone. Anything that radiates that sweet, hypnotic glow associated with sitcoms, reality shows, texting, and e-mails.

We don't have to turn them off forever, but a critical part of a healthy lifestyle is moderating screen time, and most kids get more than seven hours per day[12]. The American Academy of Pediatrics recommends two hours or less.

{ *Is the TV* **"always on"** *for background noise?* ***How about a radio station instead?***

Let's talk about our trip to the Island of Healthy Living again. First of all, as the captain of the ship, or pilot of the plane, parents need to focus on navigation, which means we need to turn off our own devices. I don't want the pilot of any plane I fly on texting or watching a movie, and your kids don't want their pilot doing it either.

## TWO FEEDBACK LOOPS

One reason screen time is problematic is because often we eat while we're watching TV or surfing the Internet. Picture me typing away on the computer with a snack bag open on my desk. Since eating involves another giant feedback loop, if I'm paying attention to what's on the computer screen, then I'm not listening to my body telling me that I don't need the next five servings of Cheesy Wonder Sticks. Logging lots of hours in screen time at the same time that I'm eating will be exponentially damaging. Not only am I sedentary, but I'm cramming in excess calories too. The body gives a signal to us that it's hungry, sometimes via our stomachs growling or that gnawing empty feeling in our middles or sometimes just by making it difficult to concentrate until we get our blood sugar back up. When we're not hungry, or when we're satiated, the body gives another signal.

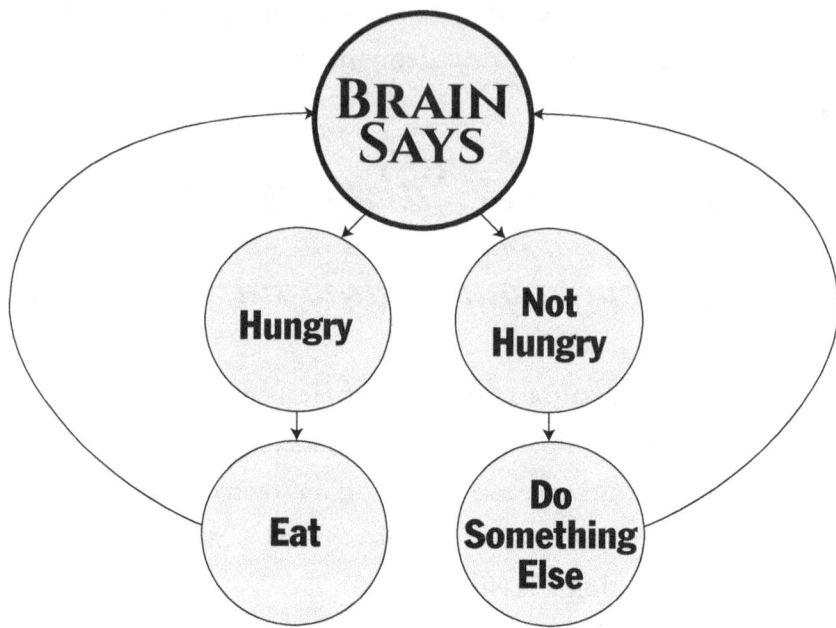

A child gets the same hunger signal as an adult gets and goes searching, or whining, for food to relieve the sensation. He eats, and as he eats, his stomach stretches out and sends a notice to the brain that the body isn't hungry anymore. Stomach good, pancreas good, enzymes activated, blood sugar going up. At that point, the child would be okay if he stopped eating; he won't feel hungry anymore. But if his brain is busy paying attention to whatever electronic device is on display, it won't hear the message sent from the stomach, and if that happens multiple times, it literally becomes a huge problem. As the stomach is repeatedly distended, it resets the feed-back loop to signal fullness or satiety only *after* it is over-distended. The child will have to eat more the next time around, even if he's sitting at the dinner table with the TV off, to get to the false "full" feeling created by the previous stomach distention.

## BREAST-FEEDING AND OBESITY:

One of the reasons breast-feeding probably decreases the risk for obesity is that a mother's milk supply naturally mimics a baby's stomach volume as opposed to a standard 2-ounce bottle of formula. Bottle-fed babies often get 2 ounces of food even when their bellies are an eighth of the volume.

The concept of over-distending the stomach is one used in crash diets. The advice goes something like this: drink two large glasses of water before eating dinner. It works in theory, and in real life it helps us lose weight if we also decrease the amount of food we eat. But if we drink two glasses of water and, in addition, eat the same platter-sized serving we're accustomed to, we just made the problem of over-distention worse. If we don't ever decrease the amount of water and or food we put in our bellies, our stomachs will always trigger satiety at excessive volumes. Since no one I know continues drinking two glasses of water prior to meals for longer than, oh, say two weeks, the crash diet does what its name predicts.

The acknowledgment of over-distending the stomach is also behind the timeless advice of eating slowly. A recent study showed that people who chew more times per mouthful[13] usually weigh less. Imagine smaller portion sizes and two-hour meals. If we take enough time between bites, we can let our mouths (and our forks) catch up with what our stomachs are signaling our brains. Of course, two-hour meals aren't always possible or practical, but imagine for a minute what one would be like and how different that meal would be from one that occurs while we're sitting in front of a 30-minute sitcom.

Problems with screen time aren't always inherent in the screen time itself. For instance, one problem is what a child is not doing when watching a screen: being active. I love the marketing idea of interactive exercise games and videos that are used with the television, but from a practical standpoint I don't see kids using them for very long at a time, or very consistently. They're a neat present in December, but by the time spring break rolls around, most kids have moved on to other (more sedentary) forms of entertainment. The idea of increasing activity levels is what the game companies hoped to capitalize on but haven't yet fully realized. I would also point out that the motivation of the game companies is not to improve health as a primary goal, but rather to sell more games, so they have little interest in decreasing screen time.

# ALERT!!!

As your child has less screen time, she will become more active. When she's more active, she'll have an increased appetite.

Now is the time to consider changing the types of snacks she eats when she's hungry! See Chapter Five for what's on her plate.

Don't sabotage the hard work you've done to decrease screen time by making nutrition goals more difficult to reach.

As children decrease screen time and become more active, they want less screen time. The less time they're in front of the TV or computer, the more interactive they are with their families (maybe at first only to whine, "I'm bored"). In theory, they will also exercise more. The more they exercise, the more they want to exercise and the less they want to watch TV. In just two weeks, there can be significant changes in energy and happiness as a result of altering a single habit!

I have a few patients with weight problems who are absolutely addicted to books, and their parents can't get them up and moving because they're reading so much. That is not the typical child, but for that handful, they're using the books as a type of "screen time," which should emphasize the point that screen time isn't inherently bad. I mean, who could argue that books are bad for kids? Yet there are some who just will not exercise because they're reading too much!

## TWEAKING THE MESSAGE

If we tell our kids "Don't do this" or "Stop doing that" (or any other negative command on a regular basis), they will stop listening to us and likely develop negative attitudes themselves. Effective parents give their children about four positive comments for every one negative comment said every day. For every "Stop it," there are three more "Good jobs!" or the equivalent. Because of what I'll call the "positive principle" (I just made that term up... don't go looking for it), when we decrease our children's screen time, it's going to be more effective and more enjoyable if we replace the screen time with something else. For the first weeks and months of change, we shouldn't simply walk over to the remote and click the red button. We also can't sit in our recliners and grumble, "Go outside and play!" We have to grab a jump rope or a soccer ball and engage in activities with our kids away from the screen time. We have to keep actively guiding play until they have the habit of less screen time ingrained and can pick up the literal or virtual ball.

## TV IN THE BEDROOM

Where kids watch TV is important to consider as well. A TV in the bedroom significantly increases the amount of hours (up to nine extra hours a week) that a child spends on screen time and has also been correlated with

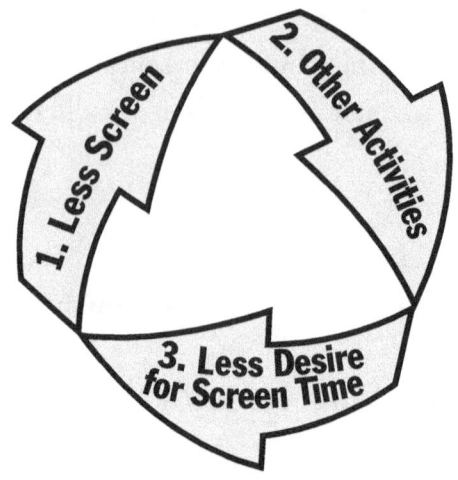

a decline in school performance. It may also increase the chance that teens will use cigarettes,[14] and TV before bed affects melatonin levels and messes up the sleep cycle.

| TV IN THE BEDROOM |
| --- |
| Disrupts a child's natural sleep cycle. |
| Exposes the child to potentially scary or disturbing images and thoughts. |
| Disrupts the family unit (parents are less involved). |
| Risks lower grades in school. |

For those reasons, if there's a TV in the bedroom, get it out. (And if your child has problems sleeping, the first thing to do is turn off the TV for one to two hours before bedtime.) The immediate response I often get when I suggest removing a TV from the bedroom is that the only thing the kids are allowed to watch are cartoons, or parent-selected DVDs. But kids often need debriefing even after cartoons, and a parent can't do that effectively without watching the cartoon with the child.

I bought a Peter and the Wolf DVD not long ago for my young children

---

[14] *Pediatrics* 125, no. 4 (2010): 756-67. .

and set them up in the living room to watch it while I went to my office in the back of the house to finish some work. I hadn't watched the video, but how bad could it be? We'd already heard the David Bowie orchestral version on iTunes, and the kids knew the story. I hit play and went back to organize a pile of paperwork. Twenty minutes later I had two hysterical children in my office sobbing about the duck and the wolf. (Spoiler alert.)

"You knew the duck got eaten," I said.

"But the wolf had red eyes!"

I lost lots more time comforting the kids because of what they saw on a fairly benign video compared with what I gained in time "alone." If I had been watching the DVD with them I could have sensed their discomfort, reassured them that the wolf wasn't real, or even fast-forwarded through the part where the duck becomes nothing but feathers. The kids could have cuddled against me and thrown the afghan over their heads and looked up again when it was over. There were lots of ways I could have avoided hysterical fear and a few nightmares. But I wasn't proactive because I wanted to use the TV as a babysitter for a while and get my own work done. The same type of unmonitored TV watching occurs in a child's bedroom.

| DOES YOUR CHILD HAVE: |
| --- |
| Sleep problems? |
| Weight problems? |
| Attitude problems? |
| School problems? |
| **First step to fix the problems: Get the TV out of the bedroom!** |

The computer is another no-no in your child's bedroom, or really anywhere other than a common area where the use can be monitored by you. It has so much potential to allow harm that it has to be in a centralized location. Don't get me wrong – I don't think your baby can be protected from everything for the rest of his life, but during developmental years (teens are still developing), your job is to protect him. Social media alone constitutes a risk for bullying, predators, and exposure to inappropriate images. Children have to be shepherded through that minefield. Yes, they need to learn social media, including the risks, benefits, and etiquette associated with it. They shouldn't be at risk for sexual predators and cyber-bullying, but they will be at risk if they are left to navigate the Internet alone.

But what a bummer this screen time message can be... it's turning into a "don't" chapter, which is not at all what is going to work when we try to implement lifestyle changes. It's like we're saying, "Hey kids, we're going

## WHAT COULD WE DO WITH AN EXTRA
# 2,190 HOURS A YEAR?

The time gained from decreasing screen time* can be used to:

Climb a mountain.

Walk 6,570 miles.

Play 8,760 games of Uno.

Get all the homework done.

Cook supper together every night.

Weed the garden!!! (This is focused specifically at my kids.)

*estimating six hours/day saved

to this cool island to live, but you aren't allowed to do anything fun there." Think how often people have said, "You shouldn't do..." this or that in your life. How well did that work in keeping you from doing those things? Probably not at all, or at least not permanently. Since I was that child who when told to stand still would make my big toe wiggle, I get it. (Don't tell me what to do, buddy.) In order to engage our families and get "buy-in" on reducing screen time, we have to turn the change into something positive.

# RECONNECTING WITH THE ONES WE LOVE

Because we're talking about lifestyle, not just weight, and because part of a healthy lifestyle is interacting with loved ones, decreasing screen time will likely strengthen family and the infrastructure that keeps a child healthy. People live long lives in cultures where meals are eaten with families, with neighbors, and with the community. Those are not meals (barring a few NFL games throughout the year) that can happen with the TV on. Consider a dynamic dinner conversation with debates about the

| COMPUTER IN THE BEDROOM: |
| --- |
| Risk for social media misuse. |
| Risk for exposure to bullying and sexual predators. |
| Exposure to disturbing images and events. |

current legislation in front of Congress. Or one that allows each family member (even the 3-year-old) to give a brief description of the highs and lows of his day. Compared with watching television when eating dinner, which is very much a one-way conversation (viewers are on the receiving end of the discourse), conversation with dinner has the potential to build relationships and self-esteem, while allowing children to express themselves verbally.

## MAKE IT A REWARD

One method of turning this issue into a positive is by making screen time a reward to start with. A great method shared by one parent in my office: for every minute her children spend in physical activity, they earn a minute of screen time. That gets around the concern raised by yet another study that said decreasing TV time does not increase exercise time. I'm not sure I believe the study anyhow. I mean, unless the kids are sleeping, it's hard to not increase activity when screen time goes down. By making screen time a positive reward, the exercise is automatically increased. Patients who use this technique have great success, so much so that the screen time is decreased way below the two-hour limit. The more time the kids spend outside and active, the more time they want to spend outside and active. Again, it's a self-fulfilling prophecy.

## USING TECHNOLOGY TO LIMIT TECHNOLOGY

Other parents have purchased various devices and token systems, gadgets really, to limit TV time. Some are bulky and inconvenient, and others are easily bypassed. Still, they are tools to help, and they require more steps for someone to take in order to get to screen time.

Limiting access to the Internet can be achieved by a blocking app called Freedom, which sounds incredibly attractive to me considering the array of online distractions I'm faced with when I'm working. Next time I go on the Internet, in about 15 seconds, I'm downloading it.

There are some of us who might say,
*"Who in the world needs a gadget to decrease screen time? Just use the off button!"*
But gadgets work for some of us. There are plenty of them too. Some are more cumbersome, some easier to use. If nothing else, they may *make turning off the TV more fun,* and less of the parent's fault.

# GET REAL:
## PRACTICAL STEPS FOR CHANGE

When you implement the two hours or less of screen time a day, remember that slow change is more sustainable. Some parents have followed the advice of Bill Harley's song "Dad Threw the TV Out the Window," but that's probably not practical, and anything extreme is likely to be short-lived as well.

If your long-term goal is to have your family watch TV only on rare weekends, your first goal still may be to simply have one family dinner a week at the kitchen table together. Or if you're already having family dinners, your first goal might be to have a "checkpoint" for cell phones and other technology. All phones and games will go into a basket and can't be used until dinner is done. Twenty minutes without texting. It's possible. If you're moving to the Island of Healthy Living, there's lots of pretty scenery along the way for you and your kids to see. Might as well look at that instead of watching The Pirates of Penzance for the two hundredth time.

---

## METHODS TO DECREASE SCREEN TIME

### Earn the time!!!
Set a timer, and for every minute your child spends outside, or active inside the house, he "earns" a minute of screen time.

### Lose the time!!!
Set a timer. Every time the TV is on, the timer is clicking. When it marks two hours, screen time is done.

### Family dinners!
Turn off the TV and computer during mealtime.
Have a basket to "check-in" cell phones.

### Limit bedtime TV.
Use audio books instead of TV to entertain your child but still help him "wind down."

---

## SAMPLE SCHEDULE

- **Current:** *8 hours of screen time per day*
- **Intermediate goal:** *5 hours of screen time per day*
- **Long-term goal:** Two hours or less of screen time per day

*MAKE YOUR OWN SCHEDULE!*
*Current screen time (Week 0):*
*Mid-range goal (by Week 3):*
*Long-term goal (by Week 7):*

**Week 0: Grab an index card and write down how many hours your child spends watching TV, playing video games, using the computer, or using the Smartphone.** That is the number you'll write on your index goal card for the current number. It will be clear very quickly how insidious the screen time habit is for many of us, and part of a having a healthy lifestyle is having an intentional lifestyle. We should bristle at the idea that two minutes of texting here and there can add up to an hour without our realizing it! If we want to spend an hour texting, that's fine, we can have that intention. But if we really wanted to learn a new hobby or memorize the periodic table of elements and just don't have enough time, then that hour spent texting in little increments is not fine at all!

When you account for all the hours of TV, go ahead and make a list of programs your child watches, and list them in order from favorite to least favorite show.

**Week 1:** Turn off the TV at mealtimes. This will be easy to do if you eat together as a family, but if you eat in "shifts" because of different schedules, everyone will have to be respectful of the other person's mealtime and turn off the TV while someone else is eating.

This is as good a time as any to start eating at a table again instead of in the car or on the couch, or while standing up at the kitchen counter before you run out the door for the next appointment. Pull up a chair. Sit down, and listen to yourself chew!

**Week 2:** Take the TV out of the bedroom. Don't just unplug it. Take it out. (If you've already taken the TV out, or if you never had a TV in the bedroom to start with, bravo! Instead, mark off one TV show from your list. Take the least favorite show on the list, and keep the TV off during that time.)

*Before Week 3, check in! If you're on track, keep going. If you haven't been totally successful yet, or if your kids are still miserable, crying and whining about no TV in the bedroom, just hold steady for a while and don't make any other changes yet.*

**Week 3:** Take away 30 minutes of video games/computer or another least favorite TV show each day. This is where you'll need a timer to track the computer and video game time, and for this use, it's easiest to "count up." So start the timer every time your child sits down to play a game, and when you get to a half hour less than the current rate, let him know that the time is up for the day!

**Week 4:** Limit screen time before bed. Replace any screen time for the hour and a half before bed with something else – board games, books on tape, or reading together.

**Week 5:** Spend the time in the mornings getting ready for school and work without the TV on.

**Week 6:** Limit total TV time to one hour daily and total computer or video game time to one hour daily and you've made it to the two-hour-or-less limit!

*Before Week 7, check in! You should have reached your long-term goal! If not, it's okay, don't get upset; just start back at the week you need to work on, then move forward again.*

**Weeks 7–12:** Stay focused and conquer the screen time issue for good before you move onto another number.

---

## PLAN, DO, CHECK, ACT

**Plan:** Write down on an index card how many hours/day your child spends with screen time. Make a long-term goal and several intermediate goals. Write them down.

**DO** make a change. Decrease the hours of screen time to reach an intermediate goal.

**CHECK** where your family is after a few weeks. It may mean taking another index card and writing down how many hours of screen time are used over two to three days. If you didn't make your intermediate goal, maybe it was too ambitious. Back up and make a smaller goal.

**ACT:** Keep moving forward! Don't skip the step of posting your goals. Write your mid-range goal and long term goals on index cards along with the dates you expect to see results. Tape the cards in a place everyone will notice!

~ CHAPTER THREE ~

# ADK 2015:
# Kids Are Sweet
# Enough

I doubt that any dietary restriction or regulation has gotten more attention than the soda ban in New York City. The restriction, which was struck down by a judge in March 2013, would have barred sugary drinks larger than 16 ounces from being sold by restaurants, movie theaters, and many other food-service establishments. The idea behind the restriction was that it would "force" a decrease in sugary beverage consumption since patrons wouldn't be willing to spend twice as much money to get twice as much soda. The law created a lot of push-back, anger, and lawsuits, but for all that, I think Mayor Bloomberg's intentions were good. And I think that if New Yorkers didn't have problems with obesity, the sugar-sweetened beverage restriction would never have come up. If we don't regulate ourselves, the government will, and that's about as fun as hugging a boa constrictor.

The really exciting news, and what the attempted soda ban also can point out, is how easy it is to cut extra calories out of our diet every day by just changing what we drink. It's only in the last few years that I have even started talking about calorie content on food labels. The reason? I simply hadn't cared before, and if I'm brutally honest, I'll tell you that I thought my job as a doctor was more about diagnosing acute illnesses than focusing on preventive care. What can I say? I am a product of a U.S. medical school. (An education focused on preventive care is there for doctors in training now; it just wasn't a top priority when I went to school.)

| WHAT ARE SSBS? | |
| --- | --- |
| Sugar-sweetened beverages | Sports drinks |
| Chocolate milk | Juice |
| Soda | Powdered drink mixes |
| Flavored water | |

I lived the way I practiced and tried to eat sort of healthy foods and limit "junk food." The rest would take care of itself, I thought, and please, for the love of God, don't make me talk to a patient about what they drink. Well, I followed my self-prescribed advice for years, and the idea of everything taking care of itself was pretty much true, although I'm the first to admit I love junk food and moderation has never been my strong point. The thing is, I always burned off the calories. But then came baby number three, and the big four-oh. Man, the pounds just didn't come off as easily as I had expected, and I realized that I may talk about people moving to the Island of Healthy Living, but maybe I ought to pack up and move there myself sometime soon. I also learned a pesky fact of life about metabolism changing with age.

I started looking to my diet for easy ways to cut back the calories. What I found was that along with junk food, I loved soda. Not a big deal, right? I didn't drink it every day. But it took me 20 minutes of treadmill exercise one day to burn off the calories I had consumed the day before in just one drink. Since I would rather spend 20 minutes a day doing almost anything besides pretending I'm a gerbil, I stopped drinking soda.

## THE SCIENCE BEHIND THE CALORIES

What's just as important as the number of calories in SSBs is the type of calories that are consumed. They're "empty" calories, not even quantifiable to zero on the number scale, and calling them empty emphasizes that they're worth less than nothing. Empty seems to imply some type of spiritual deprivation, something that could be more damaging, more negative than just nothing. And it could. Because the calories that come from simple sugars give a sugar "high" in the bloodstream, the body responds by bumping up insulin levels, the chemical needed to help process sugar, and that increase in insulin throws up a flare to the liver that it's time to start storing FAT. The body says, "Hey, we got to level things out here a little, better store up the slow-burning material (fat) 'cause we got a whole lot of the quick-burning stuff (empty calories) coming down the gullet right and left."

*For the next week,*
**keep track of everything your child drinks.**
Use one index card each day,
and at the end of the week,
*look for an easy place to decrease SSBs!*

That fat storing was helpful when we were all hunter-gatherers and came upon a berry patch somewhere and gorged ourselves for a day, because our bodies would "take care of us" by adapting to the possibility of no berry patch for a week. It would shift the focus from digesting carbs to building fat stores. The problem is, there are plenty of berry patches around these days in the form of SSBs, but our bodies haven't evolved yet to adapt to such a carb-rich environment.

## SSBs AND LIFESTYLE

The number of calories matters, but the type of calories matters as well. But remember, this isn't a parenting guide about calories, right? Or about simple sugars or complex sugars, macronutrients or micronutrients. This book is about lifestyle. And the question about sugar-sweetened beverages is ultimately: how does decreasing SSB consumption improve lifestyle? It does so in four ways:

1. **By saving money.** In preparation for writing this chapter, I stopped by a coffee shop to get a latte. I swear the next book is going to be about

making me look good. This one is about being honest. By the time this chapter is drafted, I will have consumed 540 calories, and I spent almost $5 to do it. The drink was absolutely my choice, but I need to acknowledge that choice. If I get that latte once a week, by the end of the year I will have chosen to spend $260 on a beverage instead of on new books or my kids' college fund, or an extra payment on my mortgage principal.

I'm not saying the choice was wrong. But I am saying I made an active choice, and while there are definitely some pluses to the drink (have you seen the way the caramel drizzles on top of the whipped cream – it's pure art), there are financial negatives I needed to consciously factor in as well.[15]

**2. By setting priorities about health.** What we do day in and day out, what is habitual, doesn't require a choice. It doesn't involve weighing pros and cons of the goods and bads, and since I hope I gave a good example of the pros and cons of at least one sugar-sweetened beverage (the latte), the ingestion of one, quite frankly, shouldn't be a habit. If instead of soda or juice, a sports drink, flavored water, or an imitation fruit drink, our kids drink plain water on a regular basis, then when they're at a birthday party or at a pizza party after the big game and they ask for a soda, we can take a minute to weigh the pros and cons of the drink.

Even better than processing the pros and cons on the spot is the idea that we'll have a conversation with our kids before the party about all the choices that we make when we choose to drink soda or sports drinks. And the thing is, although the parent is 99% in control, the kids usually make the healthy choice. Just ask my daughter. We went

---

[15] Another negative to the latte is that I just chose to either spend another 40 minutes on the treadmill, or eat beans and celery sticks for two days instead of my normal carb servings.

to dinner the other day, and I was contemplating my now once-an-eon soda. "Don't you think water's the better choice?" she said. For the most part, kids are wired to seek out health, if for no other reason than it's a good way to ensure survival of the species. If they have the knowledge they need and if the opportunity to choose something healthy is easier than the opportunity to choose something unhealthy, well, just step back and let them make their choice.

3. **By evening out children's mood swings.** This is up for debate, and I will say I come down on the side that my kids aren't affected much by excess sugar. My husband, however, takes the exact opposite stance, even though I've pointed out studies that suggest the behavior is due to placebo effect or relative to the parents' expectations. Sometimes after dessert or a large SSB, the kids are pretty wild, though, and he says, "See? Seriously you don't think what they eat affects them?" I get his point. And in theory it makes sense.

I have a whole lot of parents and grandparents who anecdotally relate how diet affects a child's mood, from red dye number whatever to simple sugars to gluten to nuts. At some point, it's difficult to look people in the eye and say that specific ingredients aren't the culprits behind bad behavior. So now I've switched my conversation with parents to say essentially, "Garbage in, garbage out."

If you feed your child high-quality foods, and they aren't allowed to go through the sugar slumps before mealtime, then chances are you can expect better behavior and decision making. That theory is certainly borne out in the studies that suggest that children who eat breakfast perform better academically.[16] On the other hand, if your child's blood sugar is equivalent to a ride on Space Mountain, he's going to have some ups and downs emotionally and from a behavior standpoint as well.

[16] *Journal of the American Dietetic Association* 105 (2005): 743-60.

**4. By saving our smiles.** Dentists everywhere will get behind me on this, and the sad thing is that we see the effects of this often before a child is 2 years old, sometimes sooner when the kids have baby bottle tooth decay. Their teeth are rotten with very little besides pulp remaining to chew their snacks at day care. The destruction that happens in bottle tooth caries is the same thing that happens to kids' teeth in elementary school and up – the bacteria that normally live in the mouth do happy dances every time they get sugar, and while they do happy dances, their tap-dancing feet are eroding the enamel of kids' teeth.

I don't know a lot of parents who are willing to feed their kids a sports drink and then whip out the toothbrush and toothpaste at the side of the basketball court, but the other option is to let that sugar sit there and cause decay. The recommendation for brushing teeth three times daily came with the idea of brushing after meals. But if our kids are drinking sugar all day, they should be in perma-brush mode! Which, of course, is impossible.

## SUGAR SUBSTITUTES AND BATTERY ACID

I often hear parents say the SSB rule doesn't apply to them because the family only drinks diet soda or flavored water, or water with a tiny bit of juice for flavoring. In and of themselves, the diet sodas aren't bad as far as calories go, but they change the fluid that a child mentally associates with quenching thirst. Ultimately, the child seeks out those tastes in other places, and it becomes almost impossible for the child to not drink SSBs. Which is why studies suggest that children will gain weight when they drink diet beverages.[17] How unfair is that? The calories aren't zero, they're Potential.

[17] Sharon P. Fowler, Ken Williams, Roy G. Resendez, Kelly J. Hunt, Helen P. Hazuda, and Michael P. Stern, "Fueling the Obesity Epidemic? Artificially Sweetened Beverage Use and Long-Term Weight Gain," Obesity 16, no. 8 (2008): 1894-1900.

| FOODS WITH HIGH WATER CONTENT | | |
|---|---|---|
| Soups | Cucumbers | Watermelons |
| Cantaloupes | Strawberries | Blueberries |
| Lettuce | Yogurt | Pineapple |

What about the child who refuses to drink water? Well, if the child is developmentally normal, I would argue that the refusal is a behavior pattern, not a deal breaker on the willingness-to-live scale. And the parental response that will overcome that refusal is to offer only water as a beverage, but offer it with love instead of tyranny. Now, it may be kinder and gentler to wean the child down; for instance, week one he gets 3/4 juice and 1/4 water, week two is 1/2 and 1/2, week three is 1/4 juice and 3/4 water, etc. But one day there will be only water in the cup, and if your child throws it across the table and screams, "NO!" the answer is not to pick it up and refill it with juice. If you're worried that you have the super strong-willed child who will hold out for the juice flavor in his drink as opposed to staying alive, just keep the water available, don't give in to the juice tantrum, and make sure to serve foods with a high water content to prevent dehydration.

A final argument against soda is the amount of chemicals in the drink. If you can't understand what's on the label, why would you put it in your body? To be more graphic, why would someone want to ingest the equivalent of battery acid or embalming fluid? Most of us can't pronounce the preservatives in the drinks, much less give a coherent response to the question of how they affect our kids. One chemical, calcium carbonate, may actually decrease the ability to absorb calcium and may increase the chances that teenage girls will develop more fragile bones than girls who don't drink carbonated beverages. Which is why sparkly water is one step above soda on the health scale, but probably not by much. A person drinking lots of soda has to acknowledge her choice – to sacrifice her kidneys and/or liver and/or stomach lining because of the chemicals in the drink to give a very short-term gratification to her taste buds.

What does a body need? Water. And when our kids are thirsty, we shouldn't be giving them a meal in a cup. We should be giving them what they are begging for: water!

I had a surreal experience the other day when I purchased some bottled water and I read the label. Sodium was added for taste! What??? I wanted water. And I didn't need taste. But that's how disordered our drinking has become when our bottled water needs additives.

## GET REAL: PRACTICAL STEPS FOR CHANGE

The goal is to be healthier, not to be perfect. First, you need a good idea of how many sugar-sweetened beverages your child consumes, so keep track for a week before you set your goal. Quite frankly, the goal probably shouldn't be to abstain totally from sugar-sweetened beverages. Do you really want your child to be the only one at the bar mitzvah who turns down the punch and says he can only drink water? Of course not! What I would expect is to aim for moderation, and – everyone say it together now – a healthy lifestyle.

After you've tracked the amount of SSBs your child drinks, decide on your long-term goal and write it down. Once you have a long-term goal, write down intermediate steps to get there. If your child is drinking juice three times a day along with four sodas at mealtime and only drinks flavored water in between, a reasonable first goal might be to replace just one SSB with water every other day. Even though your long-term goal might be to transition to all water beverages, don't be discouraged if you spend a lot of time accomplishing your intermediate goals. Here's an example of how much impact you can have with just one small change.

**Week 0:** Brenda is drinking seven SSBs a day, at an average of 120 calories per 8 ounces of juice. She's consuming 840 extra calories in her drinks every day.

**Week 1:** Each day she replaces one of those SSBs with water, so by the end of Week 1, she's only consuming 720 extra calories a day, and at the end of the week, she has consumed 840 FEWER calories than she did the week before.

**Week 2:** She replaces another SSB with water. She's still drinking five SSBs a day, which might seem like a lot, but by the end of Week 2, she's drinking 1,680 fewer calories!

If the rate of decrease that Brenda made is too extreme, don't stress. You don't have to change every day. Instead, replace one SSB with water on Monday and Friday. Or once a month. It doesn't matter how long it takes. You're in this for the long haul. There probably is a point where the changes are so incremental and benign that you won't feel like you're making progress, so you'll likely have to make changes that cause at least a little discomfort, but extreme discomfort won't work.

The important part of changing the beverage habit is that after you've made the change, it's critical to maintain the habit for a length of time before making another change. I know that if you're reading this guide, regardless of what I've said about lifestyle changes being applicable to everyone, it's probably because your child has a weight problem. And if that's true, you're going to want results fast. Immediately. Yesterday. Decreasing SSBs will have the fastest impact on your child's weight that any of the sections will have, but fast isn't what's important. What's important is the ability to maintain. You don't want to get to the Island of Healthy Living, build one sand castle, and head back to the city.

# SAMPLE SCHEDULE

---

⋇ **Current SSBs:** 7 *Servings\*/day*

⋇ **Intermediate goal:** *Water only at mealtime*

⋇ **Long-term goal:** *SSBs are only a "treat"*

*One serving = 8 ounces

---

*MAKE YOUR OWN SCHEDULE!*

*Current SSBs (Week 0):*

*Mid-range goal (by Week 3):*

*Long-term goal (by Week 7):*

**Week 0:** Grab an index card and write down how any drinks your child consumes other than low-fat white milk or water. (That will be how the Current SSBs number above is discovered.)

**Week 1:** Replace all drinks at mealtime with water. Do not change the number of SSBs at other times of the day.

**Week 2:** Decrease the serving sizes of SSBs by half. Do this by serving juice, 2-liter soda beverages or powdered drink mixes in a smaller cup. You'll have to find the volume of different cups you have by filling them up and pouring the water into a glass measuring cup. Different sizes can be deceptive regarding what volume they contain. Instead of drinking a can of soda, pour half into a glass or purchase the small cans. When you eat out, decrease the serving size of your beverage to small and refill only with water.

***Before Week 3,** check in! If you're on track, move to the next intermediate goal. If you haven't been totally successful in decreasing serving sizes, don't move on, but work on that for another week instead!*

**Week 3:** Dilute the remaining SSB juices and fruit drinks with water so they are only 1/4 SSB and 3/4 water. For soda, limit intake to one 6-ounce serving daily.

**Week 4:** Make all drinks water except for one "treat" every day. (Up to 16 ounces of skim or 1% white milk is okay in addition to water.)

**Week 5:** Limit the one "treat" of SSB to a weekend day. All other drinks during the week are water or low-fat white milk.

**Week 6:** Limit the SSB to only special occasions – birthday parties, banquets, sleep-overs, etc.

***Before Week 7,** check in! You should have reached your long-term goal! If not, it's okay, don't get upset; just start back at the week you need to work on, then move forward again.*

**Weeks 7–12:** Stay focused and conquer the SSB issue for good before you move to another number.

## PLAN, DO, CHECK, ACT

**Plan:** Write down on an index card how many SSBs/day your child is drinking every day. Make a long-term goal and many intermediate goals.

**DO** make a change. Decrease the amount of SSBs that your child is drinking in order to get to your intermediate goal.

**CHECK** where your family is after a few weeks. It may mean taking another index card and writing down how many SSBs everyone is drinking over two to three days. If you didn't make your intermediate goal, maybe it was too ambitious. Back up and make a smaller goal.

**ACT:** Keep moving forward! Post your long-term goal somewhere that's visible for the whole family, and beside it, post the intermediate goal you're working toward.

# ~ CHAPTER FOUR ~

# ADK 2015: Get Moving!

# GET MOVING!

The number 1 represents one hour of physical activity daily, and it's the area that is almost never an inherent problem for kids. They will be active if they're given half a chance, so if you're looking for an easy way to alter lifestyle, activity is the place to start because you'll get the least resistance. Give a child an open door and a yard, and say, "Come back in for supper," and most will naturally find something to do in the yard that involves running. In fact, as parents we spend much of our lives saying things like "Sit still" or "Slow down" or "You're going to get hurt." Those phrases don't apply to children who aren't trying to be active.

| BENEFITS OF EXERCISE (Nothing About Weight Loss Here!) |
| --- |
| Heart rate up/stronger heart |
| Stronger muscles |
| More flexibility |
| Stronger bones |
| Increased digestion (no pooping problems) |
| Improved mood/less depression |

## IDENTIFYING BARRIERS TO ACTIVITY

The problem is that as parents we'd rather not be active at times. We're exhausted, we've worked a 50-hour week, we're up at dawn and home after dusk, and the kids are at day care or grandma's house, or at play rehearsal or wherever, until the bitter end of the day, and it's tough to not want them to dial back their natural instincts a little. In addition, we may live in a location where it isn't safe for our kids to play outside – an inner city, or on a busy road, or maybe next to the Grand Canyon. But even if we live on a hundred acres with room to roam, there might still be reasons why our kids aren't active. They might not get home until 5:00 p.m. and have to complete two hours of homework before supper and then spend the rest of the night getting ready for the next day.

Limited opportunities for physical activity frustrate a child's natural desire for exercise. I heard a conference speaker once say that people naturally want to be healthy, and if we give them an easy opportunity to do that, they will choose that option. This is applicable in all areas of this book, but nowhere is it more applicable than when we hear a national recommendation that a child should be active for at least one hour a day. "Seriously?" That's what I wanted to say when I read it, and to be honest, it seemed ludicrous that it should be incorporated into the ADK 2015 project. "We really need a task force that recommends a child play?" At least that's what I wanted to say.

But if we're going to meet this healthy lifestyle minimum standard, we'll have to remove at least some of the artificial ways of living that we have adopted. Maybe our children's lack of activity is because we need them to be less of a bother to us on days we are fatigued, but more likely it's because we want them to be more successful. (Let's be honest – why else do we support systems that require two hours of homework after an eight-hour school day?) The solution isn't to introduce another artificial Band-Aid. Don't stick your child on a treadmill and punch in the one-step program for weight loss. When parents tell me they have a bunch of exercise equipment in the basement and their kids are welcome to use it anytime, it's all I can do to keep from foaming at the mouth and saying, "She's 8! Good Lord and the creek don't rise, she'll never set foot on a gerbil-maker!"

This chapter is not about prescribing exercise. Instead, we have to look at our daily lives and ask, "When is there an hour when the world (technology/school/a clean house) can NOT interfere with my child's ability to be a child?" Actually, it doesn't have to be an uninterrupted hour, and the child doesn't have to exercise per se. He just has to be active.

## THE ASTHMA MYTH?

My suspicion is that many inhalers are given to children who don't have asthma, but are simply out of shape. It should be a red flag for a parent if their child is not able to keep up with their peers when running around, or if he's red- faced and breathing hard when the other kids aren't, but it's important to ask his doctor if she thinks it's because he has asthma or because he simply needs more conditioning. Asthma medications like albuterol may open up his lungs and make breathing easier for him even if he doesn't have asthma, but it won't help much and it can come with a whole lot of side- effects that just aren't worth the risk if he doesn't need the medicine.

Signs of asthma are coughing at nighttime or with exercise, wheezing with colds or with exercise, chronic bronchitis, and frequent episodes of pneumonia.

He could walk to school; he could walk home. He could play on the jungle gym at school while he's waiting for you to pick him up, or he could play there for 20 minutes after you arrive. In the perfect world (oh, there's that pesky P word again), we would exercise as families and as communities. Just think what a blast this would be. You have permission to be a kid again! Tag . . . you're it! Family bike rides or walks after we're all home from work, hikes in the mountains on the weekends, and trips to the Y for swimming whenever there's free swim. It's not going to be possible to climb a mountain every day, or maybe even every week, but it is possible to be active on some level. If because of schedules you're not able to be active together, you can still set the example for your kids. If you get up 30 minutes earlier than they do to walk around the block, or you stop by the gym on the way home, make sure you talk about it. My friend and semi-hero has committed to not using his car this coming winter. We live in upstate New York, and I'm not sure what kind of snow tires or chains someone can fit on a bicycle, but he's decided to figure it out.

## WHY NOT CLEAN THE HOUSE?

I never considered cleaning the house exercise. Until one winter when it was 40 below zero and the kids had essentially been trapped in the house for a week. They were bouncing off the walls—literally (that was when one daughter learned to do handstands, so her feet were constantly thumping the drywall). And a week of kids inside was not good for the clutter chaos.

"We're cleaning!" I said, and pulled out the kitchen timer. "We only have an hour. GO!"

The kids started running. I would hand them something and they ran to put it away. Shoes belonged in the closet upstairs, the cat collar belonged in the basement. Books went from the back room to the living room shelves, and all the dishes came back to the kitchen. The kids ran. I dusted and vacuumed and swept and mopped like my mother-in-law was coming for a surprise visit. By the end of the hour, our heart rates were up, the windows were open (cracked at least) because we were sweating, and the house was clean. Or at least cleaner. And voila! We found a new way to exercise. (Music helped a lot.)

"Well, that's a little bit off the deep end" is my knee-jerk response, but when I think about it a few more minutes, I get it. I respect it. And I'm glad he's out there setting the example instead of me. I feel about him the same way I feel about the mom out in the Pacific Northwest who rigged a bicycle contraption to allow all six of her kids to pedal so they can go everywhere via bike instead of by car. We should recognize that on some plane of existence, people like that have already reached the goal we're shooting for, but we may not be nearly as ambitious about trying to get there as they were.

{
If we expand the **issue of activity** to our communities and our country, we could ask ourselves:

- *What if the **extreme people were the norm**, the minimum standard for activity?*
- *What if we made every town and city have* **health and "walkability" as primary requirements** *for every planning project to be approved?*
- *What if my friend and the lady who has an* **bicycle built for seven** *weren't extreme at all?*

## Turn the Barriers into Hurdles

Although most kids will jump at the chance to be active, some may be so out of shape that they'll need more incentive than a very bouncy kick ball and an open field. Some children might be so unaccustomed to being active that even if they're given the opportunity to go outside and play, they'll still look at you and say something like, "There's nothing to do." Of course, the word "do" in that sentence is drawn out into about three syllables – about as long as a piece of salt water taffy can get on a summer day – and it's said with something of a whine on the end of "ooo." The kids may need guidance. As you help them be entertained with activity, think "simple," not "expensive." Before they finish the whine, toss them a jump rope or a soccer ball, or point a new puppy in their direction and say, "I think it needs to go outside." The more your child uses his imagination as well as his body for activity, the happier he'll be.

If your child is in late elementary school years or older and he's signifi-cantly overweight, he probably won't want to be active in front of other kids. He may be happy to move to the Island of Healthy Living as long as he doesn't have to get into his swim trunks to do it. There's a reason why children drop out of sports if they aren't in shape. They're leaving an environment that is not incredibly supportive of anyone who isn't competitive. And the obese, uncoordinated children are looked upon as dead weight, so to speak. They sense that they aren't truly valued, and their own self-worth, which is already at rock bottom, can't go any lower, so they succumb to attrition. And even though it was hardly possible to feel worse, when they quit a team or give up a sport, their self-esteem takes one more hit.

| INDOOR ACTIVITIES: | | |
|---|---|---|
| Crawl tag | Dancing | Jumping Jacks |
| Yoga | Karate | Housecleaning! |

If your child is going to be active, it has to be in a supportive environment. Some of the teenagers I've known to be most successful have been active in groups (like the teen knock-off of the Biggest Loser that we have in town). Everyone's overweight, everyone's trying to get some healthy on, and no one, absolutely no one, is laughing at anyone else. Another level of that is simply finding a friend to exercise with. If a teenage girl wants to be active, I ask her if she has a friend to walk with. It works. There are studies that suggest if your friends are overweight, you're more likely to be overweight. But the opposite is true as well. If your friends are a healthy weight, then you're more likely to be a healthy weight. I'm not telling you to use BMI as a friendship filter, I'm just saying it's possible to get healthy together. Even if you can't find time to be active with your child, make sure to set a good example and find someone for him to be active with.

## GOOD EXAMPLE OR STRONG WARNING

A woman whom I respect very much once patiently explained to me the phrase "a good example or a strong warning." It's the reason I'm okay being a preceptor for medical students in my office. I understand now that even if I do things the wrong way, they'll probably learn something. It's not that easy with kids, though. Lots of damage can be done if we hold up the wrong examples for them to follow. If we market alcohol and cigarettes to children in a manner that makes those substances attractive – for example, showing that people who use those products are more popular – our kids are more likely to engage in smoking and drinking as well.

In the area of activity and health, extremely overweight offensive linemen on football teams are praised for their obesity. No one's going to get to the quarterback if those guys are playing! They're the players who lift up their shirts and jiggle their gargantuan bellies in front of the crowd. Obesity can give a sense of pride if you're an offensive lineman, and we need to be careful that we don't hold those athletes up as examples we want our kids to emulate.

## DO WHAT I DO, NOT WHAT I SAY!

There's a cartoon I love that shows a doctor explaining to a patient that the handle on his recliner does not qualify it as an exercise machine.

Activity can't be something that only the children do. It's not okay to sit in the recliner and say, "Get outside and play!" It's not okay to go to the soccer games and watch your child run but never exercise yourself. Why? Because ultimately, your child will mimic your behaviors, and if those behaviors are not healthy, he will still mimic them.

Take this chance to spend active time with your children!!! Consider it more important than a clean house, a bigger salary, or a job promotion.

## SETTING GOALS

When you set goals for this section, consider one hour as a minimum and stretch to a long-term goal that almost seems out of your reach. A few years ago, my extended family rode bikes from Georgia to Alabama on the Silver Comet Trail. It took months of preparation and a fair amount of conditioning (not quite enough for me to make the big hill just outside of Cedartown, though.) That's the kind of goal you should be thinking about setting for a long-range target.

Before you go any farther, ask your child what activity he or she really likes to do. Hike? Bike ride? Swim? Set your goals around an activity that your child loves, and working toward the end goal will be reward in and of itself.

**Just Imagine:** a mountain hike with your child when the *cell phones are turned off* and you hear nothing other than the *sounds of nature and your children's voices.*

}

### SAMPLE SCHEDULE

- ⚔ **Current time** *active: X minutes daily*
- ⚔ **Intermediate goal:** *One hour of activity/day*
- ⚔ **Long-term goal:** *Run in 2K fun run as family*

## MAKE YOUR OWN SCHEDULE!

Current Time (Week 0):

Mid-range goal (by Week 3):

Long-term goal (by Week 7):

**Week 0:** On an index card, keep track of how many minutes your child is active every day. Remember that activity doesn't have to mean exercise. It may mean walking to school or helping to weed the garden. Pick the activity you want to increase. (In this example, the family picked a long-term goal of a 2K race, so they are focused on running/walking, but they could have picked bike riding or hiking as well.) Schedule an appointment with your child's doctor to talk about conditioning.

**Week 1:** Spend 15 minutes a day walking together as a family. The track at school is often a great place to go if your neighborhood street is too busy to walk on.

**Week 2:** Keep walking 15 minutes a day, but one day this week find a route that is as long as the 2K race that you'll enter. Walk this route once. (This will be longer than 15 minutes – save it for the weekend perhaps!)

**Week 3:** Walk 30 minutes a day. On one day try to jog for two to five minutes along your "race route."

*__Before Week 4,__ check in! If you're skipping days of activity, figure out why. Is your child unhappy when you all exercise? Does it hurt? If one of you is dreading the activity, figure out how to make it more enjoyable. Have your child bring a friend, or let her download a new song for every week she walks. Don't push forward unless you're able to consistently meet the smaller goals* *first. It's fine to be a little uncomfortable, but if you're miserable, your new habit won't last.*

**Weeks 4–6:** For three days a week, jog as much of the "race route" as you're able. Add another activity every day to get the total time active up to an hour.

**Week 7:** Keep going! Find a local race and register. It may motivate your child to enter if you find a race for a cause. In our area, there are many bike rides, races, walks, etc., to benefit children with specific diseases or to help the community at large. It's nice to think that your exercise is also helping someone.

**Week 8** until the race: Continue to walk or jog the "race route," and if you're able, find the real race route and run it a few times as well.

After you "officially" cross the finish line, pat yourself on the back and find another race to enter!

# ~ CHAPTER FIVE ~

# ADK 2015: What's On Your Plate?

This number is where the big payoff is in the long term. Being successful here is like getting to the Island of Healthy Living on an express speedboat and then finding out that the oceanfront condos are free for life. The reason is that not only are excess calories killing our kids (literally), but the content of the food that they aren't eating has the potential to save their lives.

If you want to decrease the risk that your child will develop cancer in his or her life, welcome to the number 5. Fruits and vegetables have antioxidants and fiber, both incredibly powerful cancer-fighting and cancer-preventing agents. Most colon cancer, for example, could be prevented by diet changes. Same thing with liver cancer and stomach cancer. This section can impact health in many ways besides just normalizing weight.

## Finding Your Motivation

This is not only the most beneficial section, but it's simultaneously the easiest and the most difficult one to apply in real life. It's easy because you never have to spend another minute at the dinner table coaxing and threatening your child to eat his vegetables. It's the most difficult because those behavior patterns are so ingrained in us as parents and the payoff for this section can be so far away, that the risk is we'll revert back to saying things like "You're not getting up until you eat all your vegetables."

Take a minute to fill out the following diagram regarding fruits and vegetables. In the first box, write in what you think is the benefit of not changing your family's current diet. List the "pros," so to speak, of staying in your noisy subway apartment and not moving to the island. In box number 4, list the downside of eating more fruits and veggies – the negatives. List as many as you can think of.

|  | Current Diet | Lots of Fruits & Veggies |
|---|---|---|
| **Benefits** | 1. | 2. |
| **Negatives** | 3. | 4. |

Your chart probably looks something like this:

|  | Current Diet | Lots of Fruits & Veggies |
|---|---|---|
| **Benefits** | **1.** **Inexpensive.** The kids eat it. It doesn't take long to make. I don't have to cook much. It fits in with our schedule. | **2.** |
| **Negatives** | **3.** | **4.** **No one will eat them.** I'll throw food away. I'll waste a bunch of money. They're expensive. It costs more to eat healthy. No one likes the taste. Don't know how to cook them. No time to cook dinner. |

Was I close?

Now concentrate on squares 2 and 3. Fill in the negative side of your current diet and the benefits of changing to eat more fruits and vegetables. Don't hold back, even though this is the tough part because you'll have to acknowledge that there are things that you feed your child that aren't great for him. This may feel like an admission of guilt, but it's not. By filling out this chart, you aren't signing a contract acknowledging all the ways you've failed as a parent. Instead, you'll be listing some really great ways to motivate yourself when it gets tough in a few days or weeks. But okay, that's enough of prepping answers. Go for it. Fill out the next two boxes, numbers 2 and 3.

|  | Current Diet | Lots of Fruits & Veggies |
|---|---|---|
| Benefits | 1. | 2. |
| Negatives | 3. | 4. |

And here's my guess:

|  | Current Diet | Lots of Fruits & Veggies |
|---|---|---|
| Benefits | 1. | 2.<br>**Healthier Option**<br>Weight loss/less weight gain.<br>No more pooping problems!<br>We'll feel better. |
| Negatives | 3.<br>**Not as Healthy**<br>Overweight | 4. |

Even if I was way off base with the answers I expected you to write down, it doesn't matter. It's just important to know yourself and your family and know what you'll have to give up by changing your diet, and what you stand to gain. And just like Chapter Seven when we'll talk more about the specifics of setting goals, it's important to know what your goals are (box 2) and why you need to change (box 3.)

## GRANDMA ON A SEESAW

When I give lectures on obesity and weight problems in kids, I ask people to give me examples of barriers for healthy living, or what "tips their seesaw," someone always says, "Grandma." Heads start nodding. Everyone knows about Grandma and her nefarious sugar-coated ways. We know how she associates love with feeding and how she's using a free pass as a grandmother to make up for the years of austerity she practiced as a parent. But ultimately, grandmothers want what's best for a child, and I don't know many who would resist being part of a healthy diet as long as they could still "spoil" the kids. But the spoiling has to happen infrequently! Set a "spoil date" with Grandma. She can fix whatever she wants for the kids and you won't say a thing! It sets limits, but it gives her a chance to fulfill what she may see as her role.

## BAIT AND SWITCH

Let's go back to the number 5. It stands for five servings of fruits and veggies every day. But it shouldn't necessarily be just five. In fact, it's time for a bait and switch. The 5 in the ADK 2015 plan is really 5+more. During the course of our pilot, the Health Department has come up with a new slogan about eating vegetables: "More Matters." The number 5 is out the window (the old Health Department slogan used to be "5 a day"). Although for some people the number 5 may be helpful in directing fruit and veggie intake, it isn't carved in stone. If someone is eating one vegetable a week, five a day will be too overwhelming, and he'll quit before he makes it to the produce aisle. If, on the other hand, he's eating seven servings, the intention is not for him to cut back.

More matters. We get it. But not enough matters too. If your child is eating one serving of fruit every other day, you're going to need a concrete, tangible goal – not just "more" – and your stretch goal for the year might be that number 5. If your child is overweight and he's already eating 10 servings of veggies a day, well, it won't hurt to go up to 12, but unless you're frying all your vegetables in lard and dipping them in ranch sauce, you might not have quite as much success from this section as others in the book. There are also two more parts to the 5 portion of this guide – portion size and percentages.

## PORTION SIZE

To effectively work through this chapter, you'll have to focus on something that has nothing to do with the number of fruits and veggies that your child eats. You'll have to focus on portion size. We weren't long into the pilot when I realized that the volume of food my patients were eating was as much of a problem as the type of food. In fact, if I had a dime for every time a parent said, "He eats really healthy stuff... ," well, you know the rest.

Over time, we've super-sized everything to the point of being dangerous. So when someone chooses the number 5 to work through, I say, "Okay, do you want to work on portion size or type of food first?"

If your family wants to work on portion size, at every meal, your child should eat from a salad plate instead of a dinner plate. That's it. She should do it for three months. If you eat out, she either eats a combo meal that's a size smaller than she would typically get – small instead of medium for instance ("I'd like that undersized, please") or she cuts a quarter to a half of her meal off and takes it home for a leftover. "That's it?" you're saying. "Just a salad plate?" Yeah, that's it, and oh, by the way, she can't go vertical on portion size. It's not fair to have a serving of mashed potatoes that looks like the Leaning Tower of Pisa. Although simply changing plate size sounds easy, it's still change, and change is hard.

Imagine a picture of a stretched-out stomach that has to shrink back down to a normal size. That is not a fun process to go through, but your child will do it when she changes her plate size, and you're going to need to have some tricks ready when she comes to you in what I call the backboneless slump (one step up from the boneless child, who actually collapses dejectedly in a heap on the floor) and wails that she's hungry. Even though she will have eaten all the food her body needs to be healthy, until her stomach returns to a normal size, she'll feel like she's starving. There are things to do to help.

## HOW TO STOP BEING HUNGRY

The first step is dinner itself. Make sure it's eaten sitting down. Turn some music on, have some funny conversation, and encourage your child to eat slowly. Next, even if the only thing you chose to work on in this section was portion size, one of the ways to combat hunger is with protein and fiber, so just back off a tiny bit on the carb section and throw a few carrot sticks on the plate. Or, better yet, as you fix supper, have carrot sticks on the kitchen counter for the kids to munch on while they're waiting.

There's always the crash-diet option of "filling up" with water, and although it can be dangerous if done to extremes, an extra glass of water before or after dinner is not a bad "trick" to help distend the belly a little bit without falling back into the abyss of increased calories. Just remember that the stomach distension has to be dealt with sometime, and the water fill-up is a very temporary fix.

Finally, one of the best ways to combat hunger is for the kids to go exercise. See how all these sections are a bit arbitrary, and it's really hard to do one without the other? After you eat as a family, you can head outside for a fast walk, or a game of whiffle ball, or – if you live within spitting distance of Canada like I do – you can go ice skating or have a snowball fight or build a snow fort. The point is to trick your child into thinking about something else (preferably not about the next reality show coming on). As you already know, altering a lifestyle is really about changing habits. Changing expectations. Changing the feedback loop that a child gets from a certain food or a certain activity.

We all get into unhealthy eating habits at various times, and if we want to change, we have to identify the habits that get in the way of our being healthy. Maybe you need to drive past the fast-food restaurant instead of pulling in. Maybe you have to turn off all technology for 45 minutes at dinner time and impose a slower eating schedule. Even if your child normally eats in 15 minutes, maybe it's so he can get to the TV before his show comes on, or so he can go back to texting, etc. Slow it down. Maybe you have to break a cycle of overeating.

Take a minute and look at all the different variables that will affect breakfast for a family.

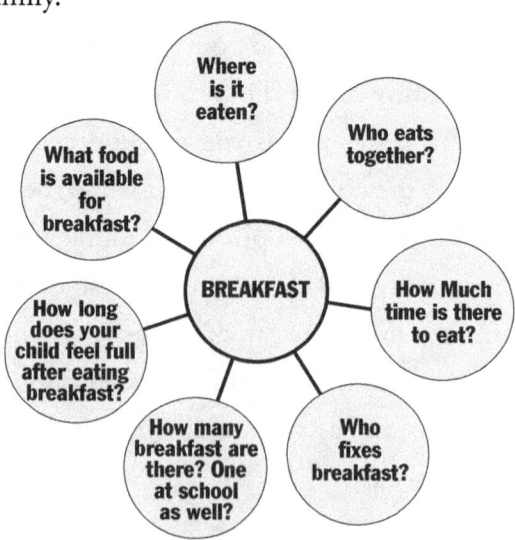

In which circle could you make a change in your family's eating habits? Maybe it's as simple (ha!) as eating breakfast together. What a great time to start your day as a family and plan who's going where when and who needs a ride and who's eating where when. Sort of the play practice check-in — that is, making sure that the middle child isn't left at play practice because everyone thought someone else was going to give him a ride home.

## PERCENTAGES:
## FIVE OUT OF 10 IS A PERFECT SCORE!

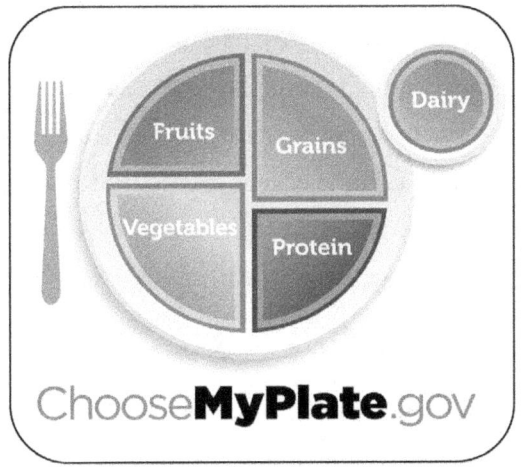

The other part of this chapter that isn't specifically about eating five servings of fruits and veggies is about how those five servings compare with what else is on the plate. The U.S. Department of Agriculture has good descriptive pictures. Essentially, a child should draw a line down the center of his plate and fill half the plate with fruits and veggies, split the other half in two again and put protein (like a lean meat) in a quarter and carbs in the other. (Gosh, I love that quarter of the plate! All the tasty mac and cheese, pasta, bread, donuts, jelly beans, cookies, cake. Oops. Got off track there for a minute.)

But let's be realistic. Here's what most of our plates look like:

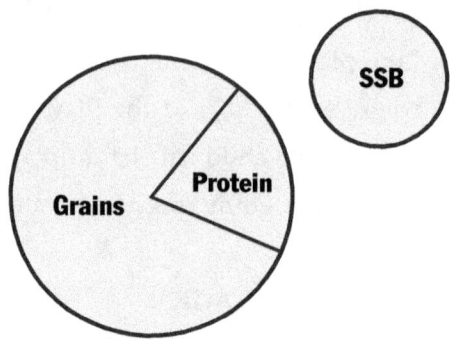

I mean, seriously, can't you hear your kids saying, "I ate my lettuce leaf, now can I have dessert?" Most parents find it easier if they cut out sweets altogether during this part of lifestyle changes. Kids will acclimate to the vegetables faster that way. Getting kids to "like" vegetables is mostly a matter of getting them used to eating them and removing the immediate gratification of carbohydrates. If a child can still get a cupcake no matter how many vegetables he eats, well, he'll hold out.

|  | Carbohydrate | Lean Protein | Vegetables |
|---|---|---|---|
| **Monday** | Whole-wheat pasta | Beef | Squash |
| **Tuesday** | Brown Rice | Chicken | Spinach |
| **Wednesday** | Couscous | Nuts (almonds, peanuts) | Lettuce |
| **Thursday** | Potatoes (skin on) | Eggs | Broccoli |
| **Friday** | Whole-wheat roll | Beans (kidney, black, pinto) | Peppers |
| **Saturday** | Corn | Cheese | Carrots |
| **Sunday** | Quinoa | Tofu | Green beans |

*While you're switching up what's on the plate,*
**consider making a rotating schedule**
*for what makes up your child's meals!*
}

## BACK TO THE BEGINNING

# HUNGRY + X = FULL

No matter what X is, junk food or health food, our bodies will always remember X as something good, something that made us feel happy. As parents, we need to make sure the first X we give our children is healthy!

This goes back to the original introduction of food into a child's diet and how we as parents often can't wait to offer that first milestone of a birthday cake and ice cream. If we keep them as a treat, it's okay, but if cake and ice cream come more often than that, we acclimate the children's taste to sweet and instant gratification instead of health. I love the story one of my professors told (I have a sneaky suspicion that it's true) about a patient of his in Mississippi. At the baby's four-month well-child check, the parent asked if it was okay to feed the baby ground-up boar's meat. "Why do you ask?" my professor asked. "Because he really loves it," the parent said.

| WE ALL NEED DIFFERENT TYPES OF "NOURISHMENT." |
| :---: |
| Social nourishment |
| Nutritional energy |
| Time with loved ones |
| Intellectual nourishment |
| Spiritual nourishment |
| **All these kinds of nourishment can be found around a family dinner table.** |

What we feed our children will be associated by them for the rest of their lives with safety and comfort and love. If we start them out on boar's meat or Ho Hos, or Oscar Meyer wieners, they will never be able to rewire their stomachs and minds so those foods are not associated with very basic, very primitive emotions that all of us seek out for the rest of our lives.

"But he won't eat vegetables," parents say. If, like most of us, you and your children have been "wired" to crave unhealthy food or unhealthy proportions, we have to add new pathways to happiness. Over time, a child (and an adult) will also associate healthy foods with feelings of love and satisfaction, but stick a bowl of Chef Boyardee or SpaghettiOs in front of me — preferably the kind with the little disc-shaped hot dogs — and you'll see how childhood happiness can be revisited as an adult for only 99 cents.

## STICK TO YOUR JOB

Chapter Eight is about control, but here's a preview: you can't make your child eat healthy food. And, in fact, it isn't your job. Your job is to provide healthy food for your child, but it's her job to eat it. You can't force a child to eat any more than you can yell at her to make her smile because "Blast it, she's going to be happy!"

| HOW TO EAT A RAINBOW | | | | | | |
|---|---|---|---|---|---|---|
| **RED** | **ORANGE** | **YELLOW** | **GREEN** | **BLUE** | **INDIGO** | **VIOLET** |
| Peppers | Carrots | Squash | Beans | Blueberries | Eggplant | Grapes |
| Apples | Pumpkin | Onion | Broccoli | | | Plums |
| Radishes | Sweet potato | Pepper | Kale | | | Purple asparagus |
| Tomatoes | Pepper | Lettuce | | | | |

# PRACTICAL STEPS FOR CHANGE

1. **Pick what you want to start with.** The easiest short-term method is to keep everything on the plate the same, but decrease portions by changing the plate size.

2. **Get your child involved.** Take the list of vegetables above and have him put a number 1 by the one he likes the best, a number 2 by his next favorite, etc.

3. **Make a rainbow plate!** Darker-colored vegetables have the most health benefits. Yeah, yeah, a potato is a vegetable, but it doesn't pack anywhere near the healthy punch of a tomato (I can hear you – it's a fruit) or a green pepper. Some kids who balk at any vegetable can still get into eating a "rainbow." If you have a toddler, sing the Cat in the Hat rainbow song. If you don't know it, ask him. He probably does.

4. **Make a budget.** Eating healthy is not too expensive! Well, not necessarily. The closer you are to your food, the less money you'll spend on it, and the more you're willing to wash the pesticides off, the less you'll spend. Cost is relative, though, and "time is money," so at some point you'll have to figure out how many prepared foods are needed at what health cost.

Take the example of frozen vegetables. Is frozen broccoli worse than fresh? Well, maybe a little, but on the bad scale, it's still awfully good. Then there's the whole concept of a back-porch garden. Last summer, I dumped a bunch of dirt into an old horse watering trough set it on the deck outside my kitchen, and grew 10 different herbs, so by the end of the summer my kids could run outside and clip a leaf from rosemary, thyme, or sage to put in our supper. I spent around $10 to get close to $100 of fresh herbs.

# Engaging Your Kids

One of the ways to get the kids engaged is to involve them, and their involvement can be at any of the four stages of nutrition: menu planning, acquisition of food, preparation, and presentation. (Notice there's no category named eating – again, it's not your job to get them to eat, only to present the food to them.) For instance, in acquisition of food, you could make a game as you teach your kids about a grocery store layout. Make a game of only shopping the outermost aisles of the store. Anyone who goes down a center aisle loses a point. The person with the most points wins a Tootsie Roll at the end. (I'm joking about the Tootsie Roll.)

Parents have to be models of behavior, both in diet and exercise. That, of course, is why all my candy is stashed on the top shelf of the pantry behind the whole-grain couscous and quinoa. Think of technology and the example parents have to set for children. Is it okay to text while driving? Is it okay to text at the dinner table? Is it okay to eat a dinner of Hershey's Kisses after skipping lunch and supper and getting home at 9:00 p.m. after three C-sections and a full day of patients? Of course it's not okay. But if I don't have enough self-control to stop such a bad habit that breaks through occasionally, I'm at least not going to let my kids witness the self-destruction. If there are clear expectations set, children will follow those expectations. Both with etiquette and diet.

I hope by now I've convinced you that this section is worth spending tons of energy on. Following the suggestions in this chapter will help normalize weight, increase energy, and prevent chronic diseases, even nasty ones like cancer. You'll have to make slow changes (change the composition of the dinner plate slowly to work toward half fruits and veggies), and you'll also need buy-in, but it's worth it.

# SAMPLE SCHEDULE

* ❧ **Current servings** *of fruits and veggies: One vegetable/week, one fruit/day*
* ❧ **Intermediate goal:** *One vegetable/day, two fruits/day*
* ❧ **Long-term goal:** *Half of all food is fruits and veggies*

*MAKE YOUR OWN SCHEDULE!*

*Current Servings (week 0):*

*Mid-range goal (by Week 3):*

*Long-term goal (by Week 7):*

**Week 0:** Grab an index card and keep track of how many fruits and veggies your child eats. Make a list of his "favorite" fruits and veggies. Give him a heads up that what's on his plate is about to change.

**Weeks 1–4:** Go shopping with your child, and have him pick out the veggies he wants on his plate this week. Remember, frozen veggies are less expensive and almost as healthy as fresh! Choose canned veggies for the days you don't have much time to cook. Every day, put a vegetable on his plate. Remember that this is an investment! You will throw a lot of food away, but it will pay off in big dividends of health later.

**Weeks 5–8:** Keep shopping with your child and have him help plan the meal once a week as well as help in some area of preparation. Add another serving of vegetables to your child's plate this week and decrease the amount of carbohydrates he gets. Keep the two servings of fruits holding steady! His plate should be somewhere around 1/3 full of fruits and vegetables at mealtime.

*Before Week 9, check in! You're almost to your intermediate goal, and you should be getting very little argument now about what's going on the plate. Your child may still say he doesn't want to eat it. That's okay. Just keep spooning out the veggies!*

**Weeks 9–12:** Add two more servings of vegetables during the daytime – you're up to four servings a day now and close to half the plate full of vegetables!

**Week 13+:** Every meal should have half the plate full of fruits and vegetables. Don't go back!

---

# PLAN, DO, CHECK, ACT

**PLAN:** Write down on an index card exactly what your child eats every day for a week. Don't leave out snacks when you make a record!

**DO** make a change. Pick what you want to work on first—portion size or variety of food (increasing fruits and veggies) and keep focused on just that one area.

**CHECK** where your family is after a few weeks. If you're still getting lots of resistance about the vegetables showing up at mealtime, think back to any areas you might have "given in." Stand strong! If you're still getting a lot of push-back about whatever change you're making, don't add a new challenge! Unlike the other areas, in this scenario, (unless your child is losing weight, and in that case, you need a doctor visit ASAP) just stick with whatever goal you've set and don't back off to a less ambitious goal. This is the toughest area to conquer. But don't argue and don't engage discussion; just dish out the veggies!

**ACT:** Keep moving forward! Post your long-term goal somewhere that's visible for the whole family, and beside it, post the intermediate goal you're working toward. Consider writing out a "certificate of completion" for your child as she achieves the various levels.

# ~PART 2~
# Building The Boat

You've read the nitty-gritty part now, and if you decided not to turn another page but religiously followed everything you've learned so far, your family will have a great chance of making it to the Island of Healthy Living! But it's also possible that you've already tried to make habit changes and haven't been successful for one reason or another. If so, this next part almost guarantees your success.

*One of the* ***best ways to engage kids in eating vegetables*** *is to have them plant a garden. A garden can be a* ***5-gallon bucket*** *of lettuce, peas, and beans, or it can be an acre of corn.* }

If you go back to the picture of the seesaw early on, the idea of "calories in" and "calories out" seems easy until you add in all the other factors that affect the seesaw. Statistics show that 36% of adults are obese, and I guarantee not one of them said, "I hope I can be fat one day." No child is sitting on my exam table crying about his weight because, by golly, he finally met his goal of greater than 99% BMI and those are tears of joy. In our society, it's easier to become fat than to stay healthy. Ultimately, if we aren't already living on the island, we fall into a few categories:

1. **We don't understand the first blasted thing about a healthy lifestyle.** Maybe we didn't have great examples growing up, maybe it was never a priority, maybe we simply never cared enough to consider educating ourselves until we had children of our own.

2. **We understand the concepts of weight, nutrition, and exercise in theory, but we don't understand how to apply them in real life.**

3. **We understand it all.** We can explain a BMI growth chart in our

sleep and we've given our kids pop quizzes regarding information on the myplate.gov website and even our 3-year-old knows the differences between macronutrients and micronutrients, and we are ready to implement and apply all our knowledge. We're trying to make changes, but man, is it hard!

---

My family still gets veggies in our diet even when we aren't feeling much like eating them. First, we pack a lot of veggies into our morning smoothies. Rhubarb, kale, and spinach fill up half the blender before we add Greek yogurt, strawberries, and blueberries to the rest. Secondly, when my kids are super hungry before suppertime, I make sure they have fresh veggies to snack on (carrot sticks, broccoli, cauliflower, cucumbers). They can wait to eat at suppertime, or they can have a snack. Even my child who doesn't like vegetables very much ends up eating more than her share of healthy foods before she even sits down to dinner! I still fill up half her plate with fruits and veggies, but it makes "doing my job" easier since I don't worry at all if she doesn't take a bite of the veggies that I cooked.

---

If the last four chapters were your ticket to the great island, the next ones are the engineering diagrams for the vehicles that will take you there – blueprints for how to make change happen. How build a speedboat or an airplane, how to form a swim team, or how to build a raft that will make it through shark-infested waters.

# – CHAPTER SIX –

# Readiness To Change

I was raised by a single mother. Although I had a loving father, he lived several states away and was not involved on a daily basis. My mom had limited finances, limited emotional support, and very little time to do anything other than help us survive. She also hates to cook, so she created comfort foods for me and my sister that cost 99 cents or less. We ate tomato and rice soup (Minute Rice, mind you), grilled-cheese sandwiches on white bread, hot dogs, and Kraft mac and cheese. We dined at drive-thrus with value menus and searched out buffets where kids ate for free.

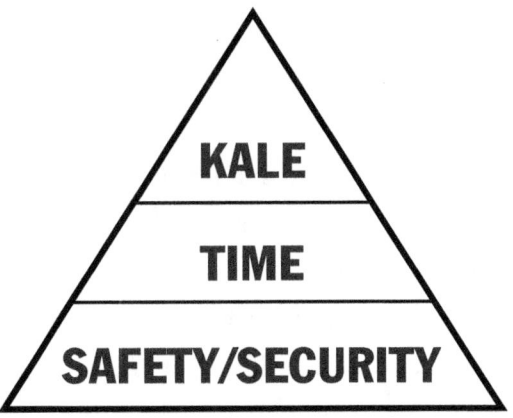

Fast forward about three decades. Now I have a successful career as a doctor and I have the luxury of raising my kids in a two-parent home. Although I still have to budget, I'm less worried than my mom was about how much a meal will cost. But what I never have more of is time. I can't buy more than 24 hours in a day, and when I'm on call for two days straight, or stressed in general, I occasionally pull out my toolbox of comfort foods and park my knowledgeable tush in front of a giant pot of orange pasta, throw in about three cut-up hot dogs and I eat it all. Until my belly hurts. Lots of times I'll grab a Coke to wash it down because the highlight of playing softball as a little kid was going to the snack bar after a win where the coach bought us all a Coke. When I'm exhausted and stressed, I'll do just about anything to re-create that feeling of happiness I got after we won a game.

# This is not about weight. It's not about numbers. **It's about lifestyle.** }

To be honest, my mom could have fed us healthy meals for a comparable price, but that would have taken planning and a level of energy that she just didn't have at the time. If you look at a parody of feeding that's shaped like a pyramid of survival,[19] kale chips are a part of the pyramid you get to only after you build the base of emotional stability, happiness, and security first. As a family with a single mother at the helm, we were always focused on the base of the pyramid. If you're a single parent, take heart, because that's part of what this guide will do, especially this latter half. It will show you ways to build the base, mostly by having other family members help and by giving up areas of control that were never yours to start with. It will give practical ways to take a little and make a lot.

Even if there were lots of problems during my childhood, there was one basic need that was always satisfied: hunger.[20] As an adult, I am 100% responsible for what goes into my mouth at mealtime. But if I get some flashback to unhappy emotions or uncertain situations, I tend to revert to the things I remember that brought me a secure feeling; they also happen to be meals as nutritionally complete as cardboard dipped in butter and salt. Actually, cardboard probably has more fiber.

Every time I eat what I shouldn't, I take a trip off the Island of Healthy Living. And I pay for it. If you think the price of getting to the island is high, the price of not going or not staying there is even higher. My gallbladder and I are one hot dog away from parting ways forever. I've had to purchase the "relaxed fit" jeans to accommodate what the

---

[19] Maslow's Hierarchy of Needs

[20] For adults who did not have this basic need satisfied, food becomes much more psychologically fraught.

pasta pots have done to my thighs. And in general, when I leave my Island of Healthy Living, compared with when I hang out there basking in sunshine, I feel rotten.

Partly because I have children of my own, partly because I've gained more knowledge about nutrition, and partly because I just love being alive and would like to prolong the experience, I started years ago to make a change and move away from the diet I grew up on. And I don't want to mislead people into thinking I had or have a major weight problem. At most, I had 10 extra pounds that hung on after my last child was born. But, once again, that's not the point. This is not about weight. It's not about numbers. It's about lifestyle. And sooner or later a rotten lifestyle is going to catch up with us. Sometimes it catches up when we're standing on the scale, but sometimes it catches up with us in the operating room when we're handed our own gallbladder as a present, or even worse, when we're in the cardiac cath lab seconds before we code.

To change my diet and make the majority of my food intake healthy, I had to go through quite a process – a lot of that process involved accepting that my mom did the best she could when we were growing up and I needed to do the same for my own kids. I also had to be willing to let go of the immediate gratification I would get from a drive-thru or a pot of pasta. I had to see more value in the long-term benefits of a healthy diet. I had to be ready to change.

Everyone has a story equivalent to what I just shared. Everyone has a reason why their lifestyle is the way it is, and on some level we know what will need to change as we go forward. By now we've seen some brochures on the Island of Healthy Living, seen the ads for more energy, higher self-esteem, and a longer life, and we think it might be a pretty cool place to live, but we aren't exactly sure we want to go through the effort to get there. We also aren't sure we want to leave behind the people we love. For instance, at the next family reunion, do you want to be the one who brings kale chips as your contribution to the potluck? What kind of grief are you going to take from Uncle Billy when you tell him you're eating more turkey than beef and politely decline a spoonful of the orange pasta or neon green marshmallow Jell-O that he brought?

"Oh, you're one of those, eh?" he'll say and either punch your arm (if you're a guy) or one-arm side-hug you (if you're a girl). He'll hug you so hard that your clavicles are one squeeze away from popping, and he'll use his other hand to rub his own giant belly as he yells across the crowd, "Mary Sue brought us grass to eat!" To get to the island of Healthy Living, you're going to have to leave Uncle Billy behind. Trust me, he's not ready to buy a ticket. He might be after he has his first heart attack, but then again, he might not. And although you hate the way he belittles you, he's similar to your apartment on top of the subway. You've gotten used to him, and sometimes, with a healthy dose of nostalgia, you're even fond of him.

## EATING HEALTHY ON A BUDGET

A friend of mine has an income limited by her choice to work part time. Because of that, she's the perfect example of how eating healthy can be inexpensive. Recently, she proved to me that she could feed her family of four on less than $50/week. A nutrition-ist colleague tracked her meals for me and agreed she was able to provide healthy foods.

### How did she do it?

- Limited eating out.
- Planning ahead.
- Coupons.
- Online savings alerts.

## Assessing Readiness to Change

Take a minute, look at the ruler below, and answer this question: How ready are you to move toward a healthier lifestyle? Or rather, how ready are you to move to the Island of Healthy Living? Circling 10 means your bags are packed and you're standing on the dock, just waiting to board the ship. Circling 1 means there's no way you're going to that stinkin' island. And no one can make you.

## How Ready are You to Move to the Island

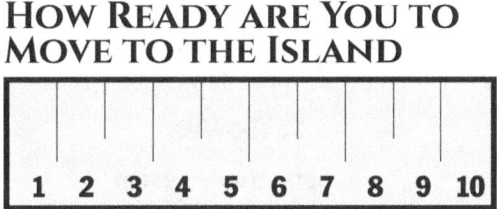

Let's say you were brutally honest and circled the number 1. (Well, no one circles the number 1 anyhow; those people don't bother to answer the question, so I doubt you did. Just getting this far in a parenting guide means you're at least a 3.) But just suppose you really wanted to circle a zero or a negative number, sort of a "when hell freezes over" number, but since that wasn't an option, you chose 1 instead. That doesn't mean that you need to shut the book now, but it does mean you'll probably read the book through this time for factual information only as opposed to thinking that anything written could possibly apply to your family.

That's okay. Depending on life circumstances and other stressors, it may not be the right time for your family to make a change. That lesson was tough for a type A person like me to learn when interacting with my patients. But my telling someone over and over again why they should change has never changed anything. In fact, I may do a whole lot of harm by pushing people into a corner and pointing out all the things they are doing wrong. I can set families back a few years by demanding that they change.

---

## STAGES OF CHANGE

**Precontemplation** = Not considering making any changes

**Contemplation** = Thinking about changes, may have started a few

**Action** = Already actively making change.

---

## THE NUMBER ON THE READINESS-TO-CHANGE RULER IS CONSTANTLY CHANGING!
It can be affected by many events and emotions:

### 1. Fear.

### 2. The kids.

### 3. Catastrophic event.

### 4. External or internal motivation—check out the last part of Chapter Eight about locus of control!

---

Even if you personally have identified yourself as a 9 on the readiness ruler, you're going to face the same dilemma I've faced with patients, only your "patients" are going to be your family members. Maybe your family and friends would have circled a 1 if they even bothered to answer the question. And if you demand that they change, they won't. All you can do is control what is in your realm to control (by the way, your child's diet is in that realm) and be ready to do more if your family moves along and circles a 2 next year.

If we rate *our own* readiness to change,
our *families' or significant supporters'*
readiness to change, and the
*resources we have available*
for change, we'll find that
*change happens when all three overlap.*

Here's another way to look at it: What if you walked into a doctor's office and the doctor said, "You're killing yourself. You're a slob. I know you ate that pack of Oreos in the parking lot. I saw you out the window. And guess what else I smell? French fries. I can smell the oily residue clinging to your XXXL T-shirt. You HAVE to make serious changes or you're going to die tomorrow."

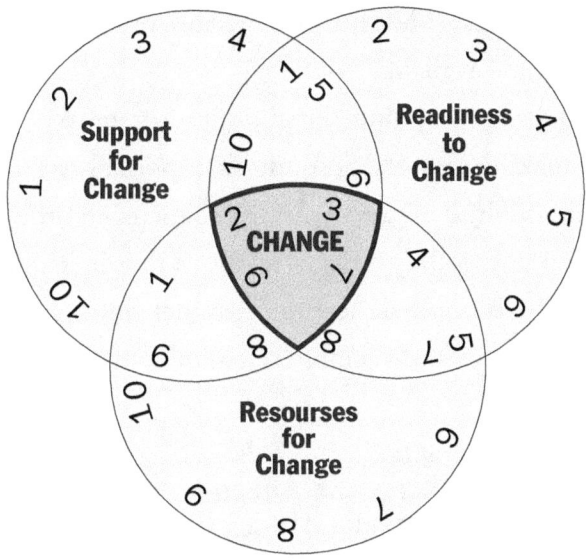

You're probably like most people who are nice enough to say, "Okay, thanks," even though the doctor has zero bedside manners. But when you leave the exam room, you'll fill out transfer paperwork at the front desk, and then in the parking lot you'll leave half your tire tread on the asphalt as you rip out of there. At home, or maybe on the way home, you're going to gorge yourself on something. Since there aren't any Oreos left, you might get two super-size meals and a couple of milkshakes and have those for supper, all the while saying, "I don't HAVE to do anything."

I should have said this before. You don't have to do anything. In fact, some things already presented in this guide simply won't work for you, or you'll have to find a way to modify them for your own life. I think most will work if you give them a chance, but nothing should be perceived as a mandate. For instance, can someone be healthy and have more than two hours of screen time a day? Well, I sure hope so since my entire job is spent in front of a computer filled with electronic health records. Every now and then I emerge from behind the fluorescent glow to examine a patient, but then I go back to staring at the screen. So two hours of screen time doesn't really apply to me, does it? Well, it might. Sort of depends on what I do when I get back home at night.

I'm trying to make two points. First, it's important to be realistic about your interest in making changes. Second, it's important to know that nothing in here is an absolute requirement. We're focusing on a blueprint for healthy living and how to buy a ticket to get to that incredible island, but nothing is absolute. If you'd rather fly or tunnel through the core of the Earth and arrive on the island via molten lava instead of by a sailboat, more power to you!

---

**READINESS TO CHANGE APPLIES TO MANY DIFFERENT LIFESTYLE CHANGES**
*Conversations with a patient who smokes cigarettes:*

- **Precontemplation:** "There's nothing wrong with a cigarette or two."

- **Contemplation:** "Yeah, I've seen all the ads about smoking."

- **Action:** "I've cut back, so I'm not smoking on my lunch breaks anymore."

---

## WHO ARE YOU? NO, REALLY...

Before you can even consider readiness to change, you have to have some insight into where you are now. I had a surreal experience the other day with my 3-year-old. She held two index cards in her hands and flapped them as she walked through the house.

"Whatcha doing, Claire?" I said.

"I'm not Claire." Her arms flapped harder.

"Who are you?"

"Not who! What!" She opened her mouth and made a shrieking noise.

"Are you a bird?"

"I'm a pterodactyl."

After an hour or so of living with a flying reptile, I wanted my daughter back, but she wasn't coming, because at least in her mind she was a pterodactyl. It took tucking her into a "pterodactyl nest" for a nap and giving her a few hours of sleep for the reset button to trigger. When she woke up, I had my daughter back. But during the hour or so, there was a bizarre part of me that felt compelled to convince her she wasn't a pterodactyl. I mean, my kids have all had really wild imaginary play during their development, and I'm happy to participate. I've played fetch with an imaginary dog called "Buzz is Bald" (who is peach-colored, by the way), and I've fed hay and water to many horses that galloped through my kitchen. But all those imaginary play times involved bringing something else to life. Suddenly, Claire was a pterodactyl; she became a flying reptile, and I really think that for a bit, she believed it. The more I tried to convince her otherwise, the more adamant she was that she had wings and the index cards were feathers.

## READINESS TO CHANGE

It doesn't mean that all the stars are aligned to make change easy.
But rather that you're willing to "put your head down" and do
the hard work.

The point is, we need to take a look at that readiness ruler and not circle where we think we should be, where the "right answer" is, but rather where we truly are. Just like my daughter needed to recognize that she was not a pterodactyl, we have to recognize what we truly are. That means identifying our negative aspects, some of our bad habits, and how unhealthy we can be, as well as our positives and our strengths. We can't look at ourselves and not see our true essences and expect to move forward and make significant changes. We're going to need to recognize our inner selves and call on that strength and beauty to change the exterior and to impact our health.

| LISTEN FOR CHANGE TALK |
| --- |
| Even if your family is a 2 on the readiness-to-change scale, listen and encourage them when they say things that fall into categories of "change talk." |
| **1. Desire for change.** |
| **2. Ability for change.** |
| **3. Reasons for change.** |
| **4. Need for change.** |

Let's go back to the ruler. Say you were a 7 or an 8. Chances are you'll get a lot out of this book if you do the exercises, make the schedules for yourself, and try and figure out how the principles of change can apply directly to your life. For instance, you might look at the section on five servings of fruits and veggies a day and say, "I'm ready to alter every meal so it includes at least half fruits and vegetables. What do I need to buy?" If you're a 7 or an 8, you'll be making notes all through the margins, calling a family meeting to discuss each number, and chances are, with a few slides backward here and there, by the end of a year you'll see a huge difference in your children, and more importantly, your children will feel differently too. Your son will have more energy. Your daughter will have a better attitude. Your family will feel like more of a team and less like a bunch of strangers trapped in a bomb shelter together during wartime.

And what if you're a 10? Well, you're going to be calling your neighbors after Chapter One to plan a community garden. But what if another really important person in your child's life is only a 2? The focus then might not be on getting more fruits and vegetables in your child, but rather on moving the number 2 person toward a 3, and then a 4. You'll understand this deep in your gut when you consider it for long. Your family, or at least major parts of it, has to be ready to change, or it's going to be impossible for your child. If they're not ready, the first step is to get them ready, and you do that by conversations.[21]

I know there are plenty of schools, friends, and vending machines out there that are conspiring against our children's health, but the biggest impact in a child's life is family. That can be a real surprise for lots of parents, and what I hear day to day and what I think most parents feel is that they are not the ones who need to change. They say that sure, maybe they could lose a few extra pounds, or they really could exercise more, but ultimately, they say the child's weight problem is the child's problem. Here's what people say to their kids (with me in the room):

"You hear what she's saying? You need to stop drinking that Mountain Dew for breakfast."

"You hear what she's saying? You can't keep going back for more sandwiches."

"She's telling you, you have to go outside and play."

The list could go on and on. I hate being translated by parents, because most of the time they miss what I'm saying and interpret what they want. I'm willing to take ownership for any communication lapse. But it's a sticky point. Let's say the child came in for a well-child check and his BMI is in the red zone. Especially if it's a day I'm leaning toward the impatient side

[21] Stephen Rollnick, William R. Miller, and Christopher C. Butler, *Motivational Interviewing in Health Care: Helping Patients Change Behavior* (The Guilford Press, 2008).

of my personality and I start demanding change, the parent may push back and say, "Well, it isn't my fault." If I say little Johnny's BMI needs a telescope to look back down on the growth chart where it belongs, the parents interpret me as saying, "You're a loser parent. Your child is fat." And if that's what the parents hear, no wonder they come back with, "It isn't my fault."

## ARE YOU READY TO CHANGE?

Just type "readiness to change" into Google or Bing and start answering questionnaires. Maybe the questionnaires aren't validated, maybe they can't be used against you in a court of law, but just answer a few and it won't take long to get an idea of where you are in preparation for change.

We want our kids to be brilliant, gorgeous, and successful. And if they aren't, we feel like we're standing in front of the mirror and being shown exactly where all our true flaws are. That stretch mark over on the side? Oh yeah, it's never going away. Ditto for the extra skin that folds over my waistband no matter how far back I pull my shoulders. But when we're talking about our kids' health, what has been shown in research, and what I've seen in my own practice, is that we can't focus our efforts on the kids. We have to focus on the family, and by family, I mean parents. Crazy, huh? I mean it's called childhood obesity, not family obesity. Maybe the name should change, even if the parents aren't overweight.

I give my patients a questionnaire about nutrition and activity when they come for a checkup, and as part of that, they get a readiness-to-change ruler. They're asked to circle a number just like you did. On a scale of 1 to 10, how ready are they to have a healthier lifestyle? Ironically, the healthiest kids and families almost always circle 10. The ones who need the most help usually circle 2, and I suspect they are circling 2 instead of 1 just because they're afraid there's an automatic eject button in the exam room if they circle 1. Of course, that eject button is only used for parents who use their cell phones when I'm asking questions. Still, the fear is there.

The families who are healthy overall are almost always open to consider ways they might change their lifestyles to become healthier. It's like they've gone to visit the Island of Healthy Living, and they'll do anything to stay there. They're ready for new things; in fact, they've been ready for a long time. And if they have a chance to do something better – even if they've already limited themselves to eating organic food raised in their own community, are currently training for a marathon to benefit children with cancer, and, in their off hours, don masks and capes and fight crime in the city – well, they'll try to do better.

At the beginning of this chapter, I could have asked you to mark the page, call your child into the kitchen, and have him fill out the scale above. I didn't, though. Of course, you can ask your child, and in fact, I think it's important that you get them psyched up about being healthy, get them ready for the big trip they're about to take. But until they're older, say teenage years, they'll look at you with sort of a "huh?" on their face and say, "I don't know what number to circle. Three? Eight?" For the most part, this whole guide is not about your child. It's about everyone else – all the people among your family or extended family or friends who are feeding your child and watching him after school. The day-care worker, the neighbors, your parents. How ready are they to make a change to a healthier lifestyle?

Just ask them. Maybe preface it by telling them you're reading this bizarre book about being healthy and there's an absolutely off-the-wall question in it. But of course, it's not off the wall, and there is a right answer. Here it is again: "On a scale of 1 to 10, how ready are you to have a healthier lifestyle?" I can almost guarantee they'll give you a more honest answer than they would ever give me. I triple guarantee it if you ask them the question over a beer or at an NFL football game. If the question seems too personal or aggressive, say, "On a scale of 1 to 10, how ready are you to help my child have a healthier lifestyle?" The risk is that they're more likely to know there's a right answer. Of course they want your child to have a healthier lifestyle. What kind of jerks do you think they are? But if the answer is 2, don't close the book; just recognize it may be a little more challenging as you move forward. It may also be worth limiting your child's exposure to the people who are not ready to even try for a healthy lifestyle until your child establishes some new habits. Of course, it's incredibly difficult to limit exposure if the people who aren't promoting health are grandparents, but it's that serious. Yes, people may love your child and yet actively do something that harms him. And when you start breaking down a healthy lifestyle and looking at all the moving parts and which areas need work, and you find that there are big problems at grandma's house or the sitter's house, or even at the school, then you have to ask whether the relationship is worth sacrificing your child's health.

## CATEGORIES OF CHANGE

Everyone will fall into one of three categories when it comes to readiness to change:

1. **Precontemplation:** Not considering making any changes.
   These people probably will score from 1 to 3 on the readiness-to-change scale, if they even cared enough to circle a number. This guide will help lay the groundwork for changes that will occur in the future.

2. **Contemplation:** Thinking about changes, may have started a few. These people probably will score 4 to 6 on the readiness ruler, and they're really engaged, but the risk is that they're going to feel overwhelmed with the whole mess of lifestyle changes, and they might

slide back to a 3 if they aren't careful.

3. **Action:** Already actively making changes.

They'll score 7 to 10. These people probably would have been fine without cracking the cover of this book. Really, if they get a few ideas or practical ways to apply some theory, they're going to be fine.

Remember, not everyone in the family will be in the same category, but the good news is that probably not everyone, especially not you, will be in the precontemplation stage (unless you got this book as a gift), but if so, it's still okay. We'll get together again in the future.

Most of the family probably will be in the contemplation stage, with a few couch potatoes still stuck in precontemplation. That's okay as long as the one lagging behind a bit isn't going to sabotage your hard work.

It's worth mentioning again that the people with a higher number may get extremely frustrated with the 2s and 3s in the family, but just remember that achieving a healthy lifestyle is a journey (to the island). You don't get to step into a transporter and instantly reappear there. The differences in numbers within a family are also only okay as long as the people in precontemplation are not the primary ones involved in choosing diet and activity for the kids. During this time of transformation, they need to have limited access to the habits you're trying to create. For example, do you have a babysitter who lets the kids come in from school, turn on the TV, and eat Fluffernutter sandwiches until you pick them up? Or do the kids get off the bus where she has a snack of fruits and veggies waiting, and after snack time she says, "Outside! Run! Play!"

# READINESS TO CHANGE MEANS
## THE PAST IS OVER

I'm not sure there's anything sadder than a child who wants to make some healthy changes but isn't in control. Usually that's an 8- to 10-year old who knows what healthy is and literally says, "But my mom doesn't ever fix vegetables."

The conversation continues:

Parent: "You never ate them."

Child: "I will now."

Parent: "I doubt it."

Child: "Well, I will."

At this point, the child and the parent are huffing mad and they aren't looking at each other.

From the parent's perspective, it's just tough to turn a hard focus on ourselves and say, "Am I ready to make a change?" and "Do I believe we can be different in the future?" Because inherent in that question is the idea that we should have changed sooner.

I see this all the time around the issue of breast-feeding. Basically, people have to be living in a box, or maybe on a deserted island (NOT the Island of Healthy Living), to be oblivious to statistics regarding health benefits of breast-feeding. Yet tons of moms who could breast-feed still choose to bottle-feed. (Yeah, I know there are some moms who actually can't nurse their baby. I promise I'm not talking about them.) When they have a second child, many reconsider the choice to breast-feed, but they feel guilty nursing one child after they bottle-fed the first. In fact, if they breast-feed the second child, they seem fearful that the first will end up in therapy one day with nipple obsession because they were deprived. So they go the other way, and even if they want to and could nurse the second baby, they talk themselves out of it and essentially avoid the question of what they should have done before.

Another example is in housecleaning. There is a woman who calls herself the Fly Lady, FLY being an acronym for "finally loving yourself," which might seem to be a touchy-feely way to talk about housecleaning. But what she says in her blog, housecleaning tips, e-mails, and plan for the week or the day is, "You aren't behind." It's brilliant. Because what she does in that one sentence is negate all the immediate responses that someone with a messy house might feel. They screwed up before. They should have cleaned the floors. Forget about the floors, they were supposed to be bleaching the grout between the floor tiles. They can't even find the duster, and the laundry room is a bleeping disaster. IT'S NOT THEIR FAULT. If I could, I would hijack the FLY Lady's statement, or at least the sentiment, for this book and say to everyone who wants a healthy lifestyle for their child, "You aren't behind. Start where you are. Forget about what you used to do."

---

# THE BLUE ZONE

We could go to the island where people forget to die. The Blue Zone is in some ways, my nirvana. Those societies have mostly agrarian lives and apparently no wars, famine, or meaningless existence. I'm packing my bags.

### www.bluezones.com

---

If you can picture my comfort-food diet, and what a train wreck that is for my body, try to imagine what my house can be like when I'm on call 96 hours straight and you'll know why I appreciate the Fly Lady. I was probably an 8 or 9 on the housecleaning readiness-to-change scale when I ran across her. The combination of my readiness to change and her how-to information gave me a clean house.

Even when everything aligns for us to make changes, there can be setbacks and wrong turns. I remember one patient who was working on weight loss and came for a follow-up visit. Even though she had gained weight, she was adamant that she was exercising every day. In fact, she said she was walking a mile and a half every day. Bizarre how specific that was. Usually if someone is "sort of" working toward goals, they have generalized responses to my questions.

"What are you doing for exercise?"

"I walk. Some."

But this girl was specific. "I walk one and a half miles every day. Except for Sundays," she said.

I tried to figure out what the problem was. "Do you think you're more hungry when you get home?" Maybe the exercise was increasing her appetite, and she was adding more calories as a result.

"No, I'm not hungry when I get home. I'm walking to the hot-dog stand."

That would be an example of readiness to change with an application that was just a little skewed.

The thing about readiness to change is that it's definitely an attitude, but it encompasses even more. For instance, are there resources available for the change? Is there a specific goal for what you want to change? And finally, is your attitude ready for change?

Parents will face the attitude issue in other people as well as themselves, and they'll face it in the form of zealots as well as naysayers. Family members who are energetic about helping to move toward a healthy lifestyle may have great intentions and yet poor application. Although most aren't going to suggest exercising by walking to the hot-dog stand, they may say things like "Starting today, you're going to eat salad for three meals a day." Or "Enjoy it. That's the last Snickers bar you'll ever eat." If you hear the zealots start screaming for a complete and immediate makeover as you try to lead your family toward a healthier lifestyle, just nod and say something like "I'll get back to you about that." Or hand them a Billy Joel CD with "I Go To Extremes" highlighted.

Chances are the passion for salads will wear off soon... right about the time the Snickers craving kicks in. In the meantime, capitalize on the energy that always comes at the beginning of a new trip. Sweet. We're ready to go to a really cool island in the Pacific. Use that energy to build the boat.

# ~ CHAPTER 7 ~
# Setting Goals

# Not Quite A Blank Slate

One of my favorite parts about being a pediatrician is attending births. The obstetrician hands me a slimy, goopy baby that smells like the ocean, and in that minute, I'm holding nothing but potential. We all have huge aspirations for our children, and we keep those dreams in the hours after they're born. They could become president, secretary of state, an astronaut, a doctor. But after the baby is dried off and stuffed into a fresh onesie, and sometime before they go to college, most of us have readjusted our dreams to match our children's abilities (and their own aspirations). We have to balance our hopes against the weighty thing called reality.

> *What do you* ***want your child to achieve*** *on his way to a healthy lifestyle?*

During my first pregnancy, I did what any overachieving type A personality mother would do. I met with a financial counselor about how much money I needed to save for my son's college. Mind you, I was still about three months away from delivering, but I had plans for my boy, and although I was flexible enough to let him pick which Ivy League college he would attend, I needed to make sure the funds were there for that choice. So I made a plan with the financial advisor and started putting part of my paycheck aside. Three months later I gave birth to a severely handicapped baby who would never be able to roll over or sit up on his own.

What's the point of that depressing story? Well, besides the fact that my son's birth was a huge godsmack to make me refocus on what's really important in life, the point is that we all have dreams for our children, and most of those dreams involve allowing our children the freedom to reach their potential. Before I met with the financial advisor, and before I went off the deep end of trying to control my child's destiny, my husband and I sat down and considered that if we had to focus our parenting skills on helping our son achieve one thing, it would be something substantial. We wanted our son to be kind. And we wanted him to be healthy. We said that last part as a given, as if of course he would be healthy. It was understood. Although our case was extreme, all of us as parents have to mesh our own dreams with the reality of our child as an independent being, and we have to go back to the primary focus we all have. Who doesn't say they want their children to be healthy?

There's a lot we can do prenatally regarding our children's health, but not much we can do about genetics or syndromes. After our kids are born, though, there are a ton of decisions we make that will determine our child's health. For instance, are you going to manufacture methamphetamine and put it in your baby's bottle to keep her quiet? That was a real-life question for one of my patients' parents. They chose the wrong answer. I'm thinking you probably won't do that, but you will make decisions about what you feed your children, and a diet impacts a child's health more than anything besides good discipline. I didn't abandon our dream that our son would be kind when we knew he was disabled and medically fragile, and the dream of having a healthy child shouldn't be forgotten after your baby is born. It shouldn't be taken for granted either. To ensure health, you'll have to pull your dreams out of the stratosphere, bring them into reality, expand on them, and begin to set goals.

## SETTING GOALS

Goals may involve how your kids make it to the Island of Healthy Living and what they do when they get there. Maybe some kids can still head to the White House, although who the devil would want to, but maybe others will just want to learn to read and hold a steady job at the local Steak 'n Shake. I have been just as happy (and maybe more so) for parents to tell me that their 8-year-old developmentally delayed child rolled over for the first time as I have been to find out that former patients of mine went on to prestigious universities and careers in medicine.

---

**I want (_____) to be able**
CHILD'S NAME

**to do _____ when she/he's an adult.**

**I want (_____) to be able**
CHILD'S NAME

**to do _____ at the end of a year.**

---

Before you go any further, call everyone in the family, your child and yourself included, for a family conference. Have a conversation about dreams. Remember, nothing is a mandate, but setting specific long-range and intermediate-range goals for each part of the 2015 sections will help you be successful. If you have stepped out the door of your noisy apartment and started on your trip to the beautiful island without a plan, you might make it to your destination, but you're more likely to get stuck somewhere else with sharks in the water and volcanoes on the shore.

The exercise of setting goals helps us shift our locus of control from external to internal, and that's a good thing. External locus of control pretty much means it's not your fault. Internal locus of control means you take responsibility. Although the first option sounds good for getting a good night's sleep (i.e., a clear conscience), the second option will help you create an environment where changes are able to happen.

Let's take an example of a specific dream and goals. Mary, who is terribly overweight, wants to run a marathon, so her mother helps her set goals. For instance, Mary should be able to run up a flight of stairs without getting out of breath. That's an intermediate goal, but even it feels too ambitious. Forget about the marathon for a while. After all, there are fourteen steps to climb.

The **one goal** we all have is for *our children to be healthy!* }

It's tempting to identify the dream of a marathon as ludicrous since just going up the entire flight of stairs seems impossible. But "impossible" is the kind of word someone with an external locus of control will use, and an external locus of control makes success less likely. Or she'll say she can't run a marathon because she doesn't have tennis shoes or she doesn't have the right running shorts or her knees hurt when she walks. But as soon as she says she can step up on the first step and back down again, she shifts her dialogue to what she's in control of and talks using an internal locus of control. Sure she can step up and down one step. She's in control of that. And by reminding her of that, and breaking the marathon down into individual staircases, and the staircase into individual steps, she just shifted from external to internal locus of control and she's in charge!

It may feel like you aren't in control of your dreams, and your child will feel the same way, but you can convince yourself you are in control of the first step (internal locus of control). Mary just had to take one step. If she keeps her dream of the marathon in mind, she'll have so many staircases under her belt, she'll be on her way to winning the Empire State Building Run-Up Race.

Dreams should be personal, and often we can substitute "dreams" for long-term goals. In our community, a young woman with cystic fibrosis made the papers recently after she climbed the last high peak in the Adirondacks, allowing her to become a "46er." (There are 46 mountains in the Adirondacks over 4,000 feet tall.) That's a significant dream, and she must have had a pretty specific plan to achieve it. But just imagine how many times she probably had to revise her plan, or how small and detailed the goals had to be. I don't know her, but I know the disease, and cystic fibrosis often leads to numerous hospital admissions and flare-ups. Often, it's hard to breathe at all, much less breathe at the top of a high peak. She must have had a dream of climbing mountains that seemed illogical to some people and impossible to others. When she was 36 years old, she climbed the last peak.

Your child's dreams don't have to be huge or grand; maybe he just wants to be able to roller skate by his next birthday party, or eat a salad next summer from vegetables he grew in the backyard. But a dream should be something that he has to stretch himself to achieve. If we go back to Mary, she didn't make her dream to climb the first step. She didn't even make climbing the staircase her dream. She made her dream really big (a marathon) and then set intermediate goals (run up the staircase) and even that was a stretch. Her big dream is achievable, though, by breaking it down into small steps.

As a parent, it can be invigorating but also disheartening to think back to the moment you first met your child. He or she was squealing and squalling and had nothing but potential. Something, maybe a lot of things, got you off course from that long ago dream of wanting your child to be healthy, and most parents cry when they realize that they've gotten so far off track. Crying's good. In fact, it may be worth taking an hour or so to look through baby pictures to recapture those emotions you had long ago in the early years when you still let yourself have dreams about your child. Hang onto those feelings of happiness that you re-create – they'll be a great motivator.

Because your child didn't gain too much weight overnight. Maybe he just had his 10th birthday, or his 15th, and you realized that what you called baby fat is still around. Or maybe you felt like you just got smacked sideways when your second-grader got off the bus crying because the other kids called him fat. Either way, you're reading this guide because you want to reclaim your dreams for your child. You need to be able to get them back in a practical manner. The first step is to remember back when. The second step is to set goals.

Your dreams and goals will be split into two parts, and I would encourage you to include both lofty components and intangibles (you want him to be kind, to be healthy) as well as very concrete and specific components. For example, he wants to learn how to roller skate. He wants to become a 46er (climb those 46 high peaks in the Adirondacks).

## WRITE IT DOWN

Here comes a practical exercise. Get a piece of notebook paper and finish the phrases on the next page. Identify what you want your child to be, and what you want your child to do. You'll brainstorm the last part of those sentences, and while you recapture your dreams, you'll also start setting goals, and the goals don't have to be only related to your child's health. Maybe you want Maria to win the national Lego competition next year, and maybe you want Peter to pass geometry. Everything you want for your child is important here because all those goals and wants are integrated with your own expectations, and his or her self-esteem. If Maria is successful in Legos, she's more likely to be successful in being healthy. If she experiences a positive feeling of control and power, she's more likely to apply it to exercise or nutrition.

As you fill in the blanks, don't get stuck by the past and the nasty external locus of control. This is your time to dream without restrictions!

Don't say, "Well, I really want her to eat more vegetables, but she doesn't like anything green." Don't say that! A goal of eating more vegetables is a noble goal; just leave the second part of the sentence off!

---

## TAKE A MINUTE AND WRITE DOWN AS MANY ANSWERS AS YOU CAN THINK OF:

**1. More than anything, I want (_____) to be...**
                                   NAME OF CHILD

**2. If (_____) could do anything, it would be...**
        NAME OF CHILD

**1. More than anything, I want myself to be...**

**2. If my family could do anything, it would be...**

---

How did it go? Did you fill up the page? Or did you end up with just a few answers. Either is okay, just like it's okay if what you wanted your child to do was very simple or very extreme.

Now, don't show your child the answers, but call her to you and ask her the same questions. If she can write the answers down, have her write them; if she's younger than 7, she may need to draw her answers.

When you tell her the questions, don't be surprised if at first she says, "I don't know what I want to do." Or "I don't know what I want to be." It's okay to be silly at first to get her going. "Well," you can say, "do you want to be a giant ladybug?" or "Do you want to help me scrub all the toilets in the house?" Hopefully she'll giggle at you and say, "No! I want to be a..." or "No! I want to do..." If that still doesn't get her going, help her out some more. Think about when you see her standing on the periphery of a group of friends. Maybe it's at soccer practice when she can't keep up with the other kids. Maybe it's in the backyard when she can't lift herself up to the first tree branch. You know your child. You know when you see that longing on her face that she can't express. Focus on that. "Wouldn't it be great," you say, "if you could climb the tree like Jeffrey does?" or "Wouldn't it be fun if you learned how to ride your bike this summer?"

It's fine to help your child create dreams and goals. But it's important for her to participate in the process of solidifying them. Write down your dreams and hers since lifestyle changes can be really tough. There will be days when you wonder whether all the hard work is really worth it, and you'll need to be able to pull a list or a picture out and talk about how close your child is to a specific goal. Remember not to cry if the person she draws in the picture is a healthy weight, strong, and muscular. Don't cry, either, if the cartoon depicts someone overweight.

After your family has brainstormed goals and dreams, take another minute for a quiz. This is a questionnaire my office and many offices in my town use to help focus attention on a healthy lifestyle. I would argue that most parents know the "right" answers, but I would still encourage you to be honest. If you have struggled in the past to figure out goals or where to start changing your lifestyle, this test will show you areas you might be able to improve.

Now go back and compare your quiz with your goals. I bet there are parts that could be connected. For instance, did you want your child to play soccer, but right now he doesn't exercise at all? Did you want your family to have a home business and run a vegetable stand one day, but your kids won't let anything green pass their lips? Go back and modify the lists. If you find a place that you limited yourself because you said the nasty C word (can't), go back and write down what you really wanted. Maybe it was a vegetable stand, or maybe it was to get off diabetes medicine or to have a normal blood pressure or to climb 46 mountains. Whatever it is, go for it!

# HEALTHY LIFESTYLE QUIZ
*Give 1 point for every "yes."*

## Nutrition

**1.** Do you include a fruit or vegetable (not including fruit juice) with every meal and snack?

**2.** Do you give water or low-fat milk instead of soda, fruit drinks, Kool-Aid, SunnyD or other sweetened drinks?

**3.** Does your family prepare and eat one meal together at least once a day?

**4.** Do you pay attention to portion sizes for your child?

**5.** Does your child eat a healthy breakfast that includes low-fat dairy, whole grains, lean protein, and fruit daily?

**TOTAL:**_____

## Physical Activity

**1.** Does your child spend two hours or less a day watching TV, playing video games, or using the computer?

**2.** Is your child's bedroom "screen-free," meaning no TV, computer, or video game system?

**3.** Does your child get at least 60 minutes of physical activity (faster breathing/heart rate or sweating) outside of school every day?

**4.** Does your child use local parks, recreation centers, and community physical activity opportunities (summer/school sports, family swim, ski club, fun runs) at least twice a month?

**5.** Does your child get the recommended amount of sleep most nights? Ages 2–5 (11–13 hours); ages 6–10 (10–11 hours); ages 11–17 (8.5–10 hours)

**TOTAL:**_____

## Scoring Scale:

8–10 = Great work – keep it up!     4–7 = You're on the right track.
0–3 = Try to change a no to a yes.

# F IS FOR FEAR

As you read your goals again, or as you sit there with your pencil still hovering over the page waiting for inspiration, I'll mention this: you may struggle with goal setting and may even avoid doing it AT ALL because of fear. What if you set the goals and don't reach them? What if you can never undo the habits that have gotten your child into this predicament? What if you try and fail and then your child suffers from one of the horrible diseases caused by obesity? Fear is a lifelong companion of the external locus of control. But still, it has some good points. For example, maybe it was fear that motivated you to buy this book and had you say, "This is it! Things are going to change!" That's a good thing, right? Well, only if the emotion is used to bump you and your family into action.

> *One goal to consider is to have our children to **accept themselves** as they are. That means even accepting themselves if they are overweight. No we don't want them to be overweight, but we know that **weight doesn't correlate with happiness**.*

I don't want to mislead anyone into thinking I live a fearless life. In fact, the more important something is to me, the more trepidation I have. If I consider the emotions that occurred when I borrowed money to start my own medical practice, I remember lots of sleepless nights. The fear wasn't for me, though; it was for my family. What if I made a huge leap of faith and then bankrupted us? Why couldn't I simply stay in my current job? At least I knew what to expect, and if I didn't leave, I wouldn't fail at starting my own business. After all, what if not a single patient walked through my office door except to ask for directions to another pediatrician's clinic? What if one day I had to have a conversation with my children about why we lived in a homeless shelter? In retrospect, those fears seem ridiculous. But they're analogous to what you're going to feel as you start making giant lifestyle changes to get your child to that Island of Healthy Living. You're making a major transition and moving, and anything that significant is bound to be accompanied by the fear of failure.

If you can turn the fear into a positive emotion, you'll be okay. Fear can't get you through a year (or more) of lifestyle changes for the same reason that the doctor who uses intimidation as a motivator is ineffective. Fear can motivate, but ultimately only empathy and kindness will effect long-term change, and that includes how we talk to ourselves and what we expect out of ourselves. It's okay to say, "I love my child so much, I'm scared we're going to fail." Use the fear to motivate very briefly, but then put away those emotions and focus on the day-to-day tasks or else the feelings will paralyze you.

If you're paralyzed already by the fear of failing, so much so that you can't even come up with any goals, it's worth making an appointment with a counselor to talk through some issues. There are days ahead when you'll need to pull out the list of goals to remind yourself why you're working so hard. By chucking your fear long enough to make big dreams and set practical goals, you'll have a real motivator to get you through the long haul. You'll be able to keep asking yourself whether you still want those dreams to come true for your child and your family, and if you do, then you'll put your head down and keep plugging along.

What about weight-loss goals for kids? Should the goal be for your child to weigh a certain amount? Weight loss for kids is not the goal for this book even though it's probably going to be the ultimate outcome. If your child needs to lose weight urgently, it's critical to set those weight-loss goals with a doctor giving medical input. There are children who needed to lose weight yesterday. I know some fifth-graders who weigh more than they should ever weigh as an adult, yet they still haven't reached their growth spurt when they're going to gain again. There are children who could have a heart attack at age 10 or 12 because of their weight, and if they can lose weight, then maybe they'll live to celebrate their next birthday. They need to lose weight urgently, yet it's impossible to give a number for either how much an individual child should weigh or how many pounds he should lose without knowing the individual child.

There are guidelines,[22] the idea being that if a child is overweight and not at risk for acute problems related to his weight, he should simply stop gaining weight and let a growth spurt even out his BMI. If, however, a child is at high risk for medical problems, or if he is crossing BMI percentiles rapidly (for example, from 72% to 88% in six months), he may need to lose weight. If a teenager's growth plates are closed[23] and there aren't any spurts ahead in the future and he's obese, well, he has to lose pounds to get healthy. But I can't tell you how much, and the last thing I want is a bunch of teenage girls standing on bathroom scales first thing in the morning.

A message about weight loss in kids can be a risky message to give and even dangerous unless it is approached with caution. While adults should be able to understand that a specific weight often correlates with a healthier lifestyle, a child may associate a weight level with self-worth, and may interpret his parents' focus on weight loss as their desire for a different child. That absolutely is NOT the message we want to give our kids. Over and over the kids need to hear that we want them to be healthy and strong, and that we love them no matter what they weigh.

---

[22] Some of the best weight-loss targets can be found in the "Promoting Healthier Weight in Pediatrics" toolkit published by the Vermont Department of Health and referencing the National Initiative for Children's Healthcare Quality. http://healthvermont.gov/family/fit/documents/healthier-weight_pediatric-toolkit.pdf

[23] Physical exams, specifically the Tanner Staging parts of the exams, are what doctors use to note if growth plates are closed or not.

# INTERMEDIATE GOALS

Let's go back to the list of dreams. What did you want your child to be or do? What did your child want? Now it's time to break those dreams down into some intermediate steps (about four) and then some short-term steps (about four). For instance, let's say your dream is for your family to climb mountains together for a hobby because you want your child to be healthy and appreciate nature and you want your family to have a strong emotional bond. One of the first steps is to pick a mountain. For instance, Silver Lake Mountain in the Adirondacks. Well, that trail is 1.8 miles long, and has 900 feet of elevation change.[24] So a few intermediate goals would be to have your family walk a three-mile trail that is fairly flat (maybe the Silver Lake Bog trail so you can have the ultimate goal in sight and close by). Another intermediate goal would be to have everyone hike a longer trail than Silver Lake Mountain but add some elevation changes (like Owen and Copperas Ponds: 3.2 miles with a 295-foot elevation change).[25] The other intermediate goals would be similar, with gradations of difficulty and length until the ultimate goal is accomplished.

| EXAMPLES OF INTERMEDIATE GOALS |
| --- |
| **1.** A vegetable or fruit for every meal. |
| **2.** One dinner a week eaten as a family. |
| **3.** "Technology-free" dinners. |
| **4.** A family walk/hike once a week. |
| **5.** Change to whole-grain pasta. |
| **6.** No TV before breakfast. |

[24] Rose Rivezzi and David Trithart, Kids on the Trail (North Country Books, 2004), 54.
[25] Rivezzi and Trithart, Kids on the Trail, 87.

That's an example of an activity goal, but it's possible to create nutrition goals as well. Let's say the goal is for your family to eat a mostly vegetarian diet. A long-range goal might be to have two meals a week be all vegetarian meals. But let's say that at the beginning, your child is refusing to let a vegetable pass through his lips. A short-term goal may be to decrease "junk food." So instead of buying three bags of potato chips at the grocery store every week, you're committed to only buying one. Your next goal might be to have your child participate in shopping and meal planning at least once a week. An intermediate goal would be to have all dinners eaten off a portion plate (yes, you should fill the parts for fruits and veggies even if he doesn't eat them), and another intermediate goal might be to substitute a meat protein with a vegetarian option (for instance beans, tofu, or nuts) in addition to the veggie section of the plate. Finally, the amount of meat protein that is on the plate will be minimal, and a vegetarian meal is a breeze, just months after your child gagged at the thought of anything green.

Make sure, if your child is younger, you give age-appropriate goals that he can participate in as well, like shopping or helping prepare meals, or one of my favorite ones – to "eat a rainbow" every day. The idea is that the foods they eat in a day should make up the colors of the rainbow. Even kids who are adamant that they will never eat veggies can get excited over time about eating a rainbow!

## FAMILY LIFE AS A GOAL

It's impossible to make goals about lifestyle without having conversations about family life and all the emotions and expectations that come with sharing physical and emotional space with someone else. Often parents given a chance to set goals about lifestyle also begin to reevaluate their family's interactions with each other. They'd like to eat dinner together; they'd like to have a conversation with their teenage daughter again. They'd like to have a bonfire in the backyard and burn every piece of video-gaming equipment in the house. Conversations about weight problems in kids are impossible to have without identifying some dysfunction or "brokenness" in the family. Maybe everything went to pot when Mom ran off with the motorcycle repair man just weeks after she got her new Harley, and now the thought of exercise reminds everyone that Mom ran off. Maybe every time Dad buys vegetables, he hears his own dad yelling, "You're going to eat every last one of those before you get up from this table," and since he'll never be that kind of father to his own kids, there's no way a vegetable is going into his grocery cart. Worse than all that, maybe there's someone in the family who sabotages dreams, someone who, in various ways, says that you as a parent aren't good enough to be healthy and because of that your child never will be either. That's extreme, but possible, although it's more likely that people sabotage their own dreams because of their own fear of failure.

Either way, when you begin dreaming and setting goals about the trip you're taking to healthy living, you may not bring everyone in the family along with you. All you can do is show the way and leave some directions so if they want to come later, they can.

Goals may be as simple as teaching skills and learning meal planning, but they may be more extensive as well. Of course, since this is not a crazy fad diet – we're all in this for the long haul – that means you might be like my friend who is a pediatrician and a nutritionist and still had children who refused to eat their vegetables. His goal was simply to continue to put a vegetable on his children's plates. For 10 years. Now to hear him talk, his children (college age) are stellar examples of nutrition, but things were looking grim there for a while. It's tough to throw a vegetable away every night for 10 years. But realistically, Americans throw away tons of food every day anyhow, so we might as well make it an investment of sorts. I guess the point of this is to give fair warning to parents that it's entirely possible that a health goal you set might not be reached in one year or even five years. But there will be progress, even if the primary goal isn't reached right away. The new Health Department motto, for example, is "More matters." Sure, five servings of fruits and vegetables is a laudable and very tangible place to start for vegetable intake, but if your child is at zero servings, five will seem like Mount Kilimanjaro. In that case, it's okay to try for two.

Another important idea is to try and make the goals positive. For instance, it's better to say, "We're going to walk every day!" instead of "We're going to stop being lazy; we're not going to watch TV anymore." Now that may seem obvious, but the second statements are how we talk to ourselves all the time. How many times have you told yourself, "I'm so fat." Or "I'm not going to..." The negative chatter we feed ourselves and our kids is just as damaging (more so, probably) than a bad diet or rotten exercise plan. So instead of phrasing your goals with a "not" or a "can't," make sure you set out what you and your family are "going" to do. Think about pulling out the goals over the next year and imagine which ones you will want to read – the ones that are limiting (can't, don't, shouldn't) or the ones that open up more possibilities! Of course the positive goals are the ones we're going to want to revisit.

Maybe with two jobs, after-school activities, and all the homework demands, it's too daunting to consider sitting down for dinner, but you really want to have more family meals together. Well, think about the other end of the day. Is it possible to have breakfast together? Or are we so committed to the mad dash out the door for the 7:00 a.m. bus that the best we'll ever do for breakfast is a Pop-Tart?

If we take a minute and expand the question we're asking, we'll need to contemplate what our goal is as a society, as a nation, and as a world. To end world hunger? Feed the children? It's worth taking the time to think about generational goals that will let us as a society break cycles and habits. We have the chance to create taste cravings for our children that are healthy. We have the chance to prevent obesity for the next generation even as we work to remedy it for the current one. As difficult as that sounds, it's so much easier than trying to fix the problem later, and the truth is, we know now what is causing obesity, so we could put policies and changes in place to prevent it for the next generation.

As another example, what in the world are we chasing with our two-income families and 12-hour workdays? What does getting more money and more prestige cost us? It may have gotten us more fast-food dinners, less time together as a family, and a fatter nation. Yes, that's a simplified explanation for two-income families, but it's an example of one factor we could consider when we look at changes as a society. (I am in no way suggesting that the little woman should hustle back to the kitchen and start cooking – there are plenty of ways to create a one-income family without putting women back into the dark ages. My own family is an example.) With two incomes, we are shifting the amount of money we have at our disposal and dumping it into healthcare, education, and child-care costs. One ginormous societal goal may be to move more families toward single incomes again and require enough maternity leave so infants are able to breast-feed easily for several months.

There are lots of ways to the Island of Healthy Living, but let me tell you, working ourselves to death while regretting that we aren't spending time with our children isn't one of them.

# ~CHAPTER 8~
# Control

It should be clear by now that if a child is overweight, it's really the family that needs to change, and one area that might be considered for change is our parenting style. When I talk with parents about their overweight child, they tend to display one overwhelming emotion about their child's health – the same one they might experience while riding a horse in the middle of a cattle stampede. They feel out of control. But unlike the stampede, the feeling parents have about their children's weight is similar to a well-marketed illusion. We could debate the source of the marketing campaign, but won't. In the end, the result is the same: parents of overweight children often feel out of control. One way of feeling more powerful is to recognize how you tend to parent your children.

## THE HELPLESS PARENT

Parents who feel out of control can be grouped into a few extreme categories. One is the overweight mother like Mrs. Carson, who feels overwhelmed by her own health and even more overwhelmed by her children's. She says, in effect, "I can't even help myself." So she stops trying, and the kids figure either it must not matter that much or else it's a hopeless endeavor because Mom isn't even trying to fix the problem.

## THE TRY-TO-MAKE-THEM-HAPPY PARENT

Another type of parent is like Mr. Base, who can't ever make his daughter happy, but he tries to – even giving her whatever food she wants. Mr. Base wants to make her happy because he loves her, and even though he knows the habit of overeating or poor eating isn't right or healthy, he doesn't know what else to do. He's stuck in the cycle and gives more food and unhealthy food hoping that she'll eat more or be happier. Occasionally, he tries to set limits, but when he does, the tantrums his daughter throws are so extreme, frightening even, that he doesn't know what else to do except give in. He hopes that one day his child will be grateful and moderate herself.

## THE OUT-OF-TIME PARENT

A subcategory of the Mr. Base style of parent is the one like Mrs. Carter, who is so overwhelmed with the business of life that she says, "Just for now" when she allows her children too much food or poor food choices. She says she'll fix it later.

Sometimes this is the parent who is very much involved in her children's lives. She coordinates soccer games, dance class, traveling basketball leagues, and a party for every major holiday. Her kids are in the car and on the road and use their home like a hotel and a place to sleep.

## THE ABSENT PARENT

Finally, there is the absent parent or mostly absent parent who is so removed from his kids' lives that he temporarily relinquishes his authority, and when he reappears he goes to extremes to get it back. I've seen this in parents who have been deployed or imprisoned. For instance, Mr. Engle was working 80 hours a week for a few years, and when he finally took a vacation, he discovered that his son had gained 50 pounds in one year. Mr. Engle was absolutely swamped with other issues. If you talked to him, you'd understand he'd just been working like crazy to provide for his family, and he would essentially say, "I've done the best I could. I couldn't be in two places at once. But now, by golly, things are going to change. I'm putting my foot down." As a result of his strict rule setting, his son ate even more, and became sullen, withdrawn, and even less active.

## PARENTING STYLES

We could align those types of parents to different parenting styles: permissive, authoritarian, and authoritative, and in about as much time as it takes to say, "Where'd it all go wrong?" we would find that the permissive parenting style is the ultimate cause of Mrs. Carson's and Mr. Base's scenario, and the authoritarian parenting style has resulted in the sweet smell of resistance and negativity wafting up from Mr. Engle's child. Mrs. Carter might have either permissive or authoritarian styles; her problem is more one of priorities than method of execution.

Ideally parents will gravitate toward an authoritative style. It's a style reminiscent of the "Give a man a fish or teach him to fish" proverb. The authoritative parents teach their children to fish. And although they accept responsibility in some areas of their children's lives, they give ultimate ownership of the child's life back to their children. After you identify which parenting type and style you tend toward, you can begin to talk about what areas of control you have and how you can change your child's lifestyle effectively.

Children have the ultimate last word in at least two areas of their lives: potty training and eating. Potty training is for another book altogether. But as an example, in extreme cases of psychological stress, children refuse to poop at all or else they poop at inappropriate times (like in their underwear in gym class when they're 8 years old). It drives parents to distraction, to say the least, and often exacerbates whatever dysfunctional parenting technique already exists.

Just like the poop problem, when a parent puts a vegetable on a child's plate and says, "Eat your broccoli," that parent is stepping over the bounds of what she should say. Uh-huh. I'm serious. Parents should never command their children, bribe their children, or threaten their children to eat their vegetables. The majority of children who like broccoli will immediately refuse to eat it if they are told they have to. But what's a parent to do? Nothing. That's right. Put the broccoli on the plate and back away. Slowly.

Short of physically forcing the child to eat the broccoli, which is NOT recommended either, a parent who demands that a child eat puts herself in a position of ordering something that she isn't really in control of. I realize (I'm a parent too, remember) there are all sorts of psychological manipulations that will result in the child eating her broccoli, the most popular of which is, "You can't have dessert until you eat your broccoli." But what happens when the child is a teenager or a young adult? She'll say, "Mom's not around to make me eat my broccoli anymore. I can just skip right to dessert." And she'll have all the dessert she wants.

If we follow an authoritative parenting style, we'll present the food (meal after meal, year after year), and we'll talk to our kids about why eating healthy food makes us healthy, but then we'll let the child make her own decisions. She may choose to be hungry some nights instead of eating her vegetables, but ultimately she's in control, and we need to empower her ability to make a choice because it's her body and she needs to take care of it. Remember we're in this for the long haul – for years of health, not for individual battles over dinnertime veggies.

This is why I think hiding vegetables in food is comparable to telling kids that Santa Claus is real and the little elves are monitoring their behavior all December. The child is tricked into eating her vegetables; she isn't given a choice, and when she finds out she was deceived, she will resent the tricking. Are there major nutrients a child is missing while she's taking her anti-veggie stand? Maybe, but she'll catch up, or (this is the only time I'll ever recommend this) just give her a vitamin for a while. If, as a parent, you feel adamant that you simply must grind up that zucchini to hide in the chocolate brownie mix, well, I think it's a bad choice and it's going to come back to haunt you. But if you do, save a few slices of zucchini, and put them on a plate so your child still has the chance to make a choice to eat it or not.

# RISK MANAGERS

If you're focused on improving your child's health, there's another way to look at how you relate to your child's lifestyle. You are a risk manager for your child. What are all the risks and dangers that your child may face in his life? A car accident, for example. How do parents manage the risk associated with that? They might drive the speed limit, buckle their kids into car seats, avoid using alcohol before they drive. All of those actions decrease the risk that a child will be in a car accident.

Risk management relates to a child's health in other ways too. For example, there may be a risk of your child developing type 2 diabetes, either because of family history or because of his weight. Parents can manage that risk by increasing the number of fruits and vegetables they buy or by increasing the number of times the family is physically active together.

Maybe it's easier to look at changing your child's health by looking at the things you're trying to have him avoid. How do you decrease the risk of diabetes or stroke in your child? Everyday choices change the risk.

## CONTROLLING THE OTHER (EX)HALF

A whole other category of health risks comes with children of divorced parents. Those children can face health problems for many reasons, not the least of which is being the badminton birdie in the game of life. They bounce between two or three different houses, sometimes with schedules that approximate the schedule of an ambassador (Monday, Tuesday, and Wednesday of every third month with a full moon they're at Dad's house; Tuesday, Wednesday, and Thursday mornings they sleep at Grandma's because one has band before school, and another has to go to Model U.N.)

Actually, a badminton birdie seems to have it easy by comparison. At least the birdie doesn't have to eat. The kids get shuttled around at mealtime, getting on the bus at breakfast and transferring to the other parent's house at or just after supper. Forget about soccer or basketball practice or play practice – mealtime is for changing homes. I want to say the example is extreme, except it's what I see every day in my office.

Even in the best scenario of amicable splits (I've seen two of those in my practice over the last 10 years), nutrition and exercise are at risk simply because parents have less time to plan meals and usually have a more limited income to do it. But the risks for health problems and obesity are escalated when the two households have different policies about food.

Often the different household policies are created with honorable intentions, but sometimes they're made in an effort to make one house more appealing. If there's conflict between the houses over what a child gets to eat, the exes probably have different parenting styles. For instance, the mom is permissive and the dad may be authoritarian. Just like the patient who gorged himself on Oreos before he went into Dr. Rude's office, the permissive parent will only become more permissive when her ex tells her to shape up and get a backbone. She may do it for passive-aggressive reasons to get back at her ex, or she may do it because she thinks she needs to balance the more dictatorial parent. At least temporarily, the kids will gravitate toward the permissive parent, and she might interpret that as affirmation that giving in will equate with the kids loving her more.

I wish I was making this stuff up.

The other gigantic factors impacting children's health when the parents are divorced are depression and decreased supervision surrounding food. If food gives a child comfort (and it usually does), then when the kids are devastated by their parents splitting up, they'll gravitate toward the feeling of comfort, even if it means gorging themselves on potato chips and soda.

I'm not saying that all this makes staying in an abusive relationship or even a dysfunctional relationship worthwhile and that all married couples should stay together for the children's benefit. I'm just saying that separate households make a healthy lifestyle for kids that much more difficult.

## WHO'S IN CONTROL?

Let's look at a bigger picture for a minute. In the not so distant past, New York City tried to implement a limit on the size of soda that can be sold in individual servings to 16 ounces or less. Adios, super-sized sodas. And now lawsuits are pending from different corners of the food industry. You see, a variety of people in charge of paying the bills (the New York City mayor, for instance) recognized that obesity will bankrupt us all, physically, emotionally, and fiscally. And they were more than happy to regulate us into health.

---

### HOW PARENTS ARE IN CONTROL

**1.** They bring food into the house.

**2.** They control the finances.

**3.** They set the examples.

---

Regulating health isn't always possible, and I happen to have personal distaste for government interventions like that, but I understand the reasoning behind it. Unfortunately it's based on the premise that most people are not capable or willing to take care of their own health. Considering the current obesity rate, we may not have much room to argue, but opinions aside, the laws are a moot point. Our kids don't have the time to wait for the lawsuits to be waged and the food labels to be changed or the soda machines to be taken out of the schoolyards. Their lives will be irrevocably damaged by the time the lawsuits are over, and some will die before their health can be regulated. Plus, who, exactly, wants to be regulated into health? For every person who gains less weight because of the soda law, I'm afraid there will be another who pushes back against the soda law and says, "Well, fine, I'll take three!"

Government interventions involving obese children present an ethical dilemma for child protective services. The question is: should children be taken from the custody of their parents and put into foster care because of obesity? I've seen some horrific cases of obesity, and I know that children can die as a result of being overweight. But obesity is so much more complex than out-and-out physical abuse – say, a parent who breaks his child's legs with a baseball bat. I'm more than happy to testify in court about why that parent shouldn't be allowed to raise his child.

Obesity is different because there are multiple causes and society has to take its own share of responsibility. Yet how is society, in the form of a state agency, more likely to be successful than a parent in making changes, and even if foster care succeeds in helping a child lose weight, what else is lost when the child is removed from his home? Is the weight loss worth it? Instead of discussing when a child should be removed from his home, I would much rather see efforts focused more on preventing obesity and providing services to families.

With all the different pending regulations and threats, the risk is that a parent will feel more out of control, more validated in saying one of the following:

- "See, there's a lawsuit pending; it's really the food industry's fault."
- "No matter what I do, it isn't good enough."
- "If I limit the food my child eats, she'll throw such a tantrum that my neighbors will think I'm beating her and call CPS. If she doesn't lose weight, my neighbors are going to call CPS."

I am not trying to create fear or angst. I wanted to remind us that as parents we HAVE control now! You can make the changes needed for a healthy lifestyle without thinking about ways public health laws can help you or how the government can take away personal rights. You don't have to join a class-action lawsuit against a fast-food corporation to have enough money to eat healthy. No one has more control or responsibility than parents when it comes to our children, and even relying on food stamps, we have plenty of choices about what food comes into our house and what meals our children have the option of eating. Even when they're teenagers, we can still affect their diet and exercise schedule!

I'm trying to get at all the things we are able to control and the things we can't, but the sum-up point is that we gain control only after we give up control in some areas. I'm pretty sure there's a Zen saying hidden in this chapter. I have conversations with parents on a regular basis about how they are in control of their children's diet (not the state) but they can't control their eating, and when we get to the end of the discussion, at least one of the parents invariably says, "So how do I make them eat their vegetables?"

At that point, I want to pelt this Depression-era-sounding parent with a bunch of carrot sticks dipped in ranch dressing, because I'm pretty sure the eat-all-your-vegetables as well as clean-your-plate is a knee-jerk reaction to a nation having been on the brink of starvation. I also want to go on a bit of a rant.

"You don't make them eat their vegetables! You can't! And it isn't your job, anyhow. Your job as a parent is to provide the healthy food, in healthy proportions, and that's it! It's your child's job to eat the food."

It makes so much sense! Just humor me, find your happy place, think in Zennish, and take a deep breath. Hold it, and as you sigh out, say, "My job is to provide the food, his job is to eat it." Repeat about five billion times a day, or anytime you feel the urge to tell your child to eat his broccoli. You don't want to be that employee at work who's so busy trying to do everyone else's job that she doesn't do her own well.

## AREAS OF LIFE THAT WE CONTROL

To move forward quickly and impact your child's health this year, you have to take back the control that you relinquished or the control you feel like you never had. Specifically: what food to buy, what to prepare, and what to do for family activities. Own those areas of your life as areas under your control! The tough part of this idea is that as soon as you take back control, you'll also acknowledge that you're taking back responsibility, and as soon as you accept responsibility again, that ugly emotion of fear is going to start nagging you. The idea of taking back responsibility is a little bit misleading, since we always had responsibility, but by saying essentially, "It's out of my control," we're also saying, "It's not my fault." That's a problematic way to think. This is not about fault; this is not about pointing fingers. It is about acknowledging your innate power to help your child get to that Island of Healthy Living.

## LOCUS OF CONTROL[26]

Did you figure out your inherent locus of control while you were reading

---

[26] Julian Rotter introduced the idea of internal and external locus of control by publishing an I-E scale in 1966. Since then, the scale has been used to identify markers for business success, as well as methods to improve individual health. While there is some frustration and disagreement about how limiting the test is, it can give a fair amount of insight into a parent's tendencies toward one locus or the other.

Chapter Seven? Locus of control is internal or external, and, in effect, influences a person to say either, "I'm in charge of the things that happen in my life" or "I'm just a piece of dust getting blown around." Clearly an internal locus of control equates to a feeling of power. There are whole books written in the field of health psychology about how loci of control relate to specific behaviors. People gravitate to or display one locus or another, and the individuals with naturally internal loci of control are a step ahead in the fight toward a healthy lifestyle.

# WHO'S IN CONTROL?

Someone with an INTERNAL LOCUS of control says, "I am!"

Someone with an EXTERNAL LOCUS of control says, "Not me!"

A healthy lifestyle is tough, and even parents with an internal locus of control will at some point say, "I can't help it if my child has a weight problem." But because their inclination is to admit control, they can change that shaky attitude pretty quickly. After all, they believe they are in charge of their destinies.

Parents with an external locus of control will have a harder time moving their family toward a healthier lifestyle because, "It's not up to me anyhow. There are too many things in life I can't control." Lucky that locus of control is not one of those things. The natural tendency can be shifted, like taking a dial and twisting it toward the "I'm in control" side of life. Start twisting that dial, even if it only has to do with your child's weight.

**EXTERNAL LOCUS OF CONTROL SAYS:**
*"I can't control what my child eats."*
*"All the people in my family are fat."*
*"The school lunches are awful."*
*"Grandma is the one who feeds him all the junk food."*
*"He doesn't like vegetables."*
*"Fresh fruits and vegetables are too expensive."*

To give an example of how to alter your inherent feelings of power, consider Mrs. Parker, who says, "I can't control what my child eats." Without much effort or angst, she can shift that statement a little bit to say, "I'm the one who pays the grocery bills." Maybe she can't change her inherent feeling that life is subject to the whims of the Fates, but she can identify one area that she can be in charge of. Once she shifts from "can't" over to the more powerful side of life, she can then say, "I'm the one who pays the grocery bills, so I'm in charge of what I buy." Now that's a bigger leap, but it's possible to begin to think that way, at least to recognize the areas where we think we've lost control, and find out we really had it all along.

## Practical Steps to Take Control

One of the best ways to begin to regain control in your child's health is to set a schedule. Kids, even those (especially those) who gravitate toward chaos, thrive with routine. Take a look again at the breakfast mealtime schematic in Chapter Five. One meal, the most important one of the day if you believe the marketing, can be a nutritional disaster and an emotional nightmare. How many parents end up yelling at the kids by the time the school bus comes because, "You aren't moving fast enough and you're going to be late and did you get your homework off the table and WHAT!? There's a spelling test today???"

### HOW TO TAKE CONTROL

**1.** MAKE A SCHEDULE OF THE DAYS *AND* MEALS.

**2.** SET A BUDGET.

**3.** SET AN EXAMPLE.

How would a schedule help that train wreck? Well, if your locus of control is typically external, your first response will be that nothing will help, you can't change any of those forces influencing breakfast. But if you estimate how much time each step will take, and shift some tasks to the night before, all of a sudden it's possible to sit down and have a meal that approximates the Choose My Plate schematic.

That's just one meal. It may help to draw out a schematic like that and show the kids and family what needs to be done for every meal. Maybe the kids want to rotate packing lunches, or maybe they're really good at toasting bread or peeling oranges, so they take over that for the morning. Maybe Dad packs the lunches, but he does it the night before. So many options, but if it isn't planned out, chaos happens.

The chaos theory[27] can relate to family life. Essentially small changes can effect unpredictable results and, you guessed it, chaos. Those extra five minutes that Johnny spends with his pillow over his head are negligible compared with an hour, but when he finally throws the covers back and ejects the cat from the comforter, the cat streaks through the house. The dog lunges for the cat, knocks into the toddler, who falls against the coffee table, and because of Johnny's five extra minutes of sleep, you're packing everyone up to go to the emergency room to have stitches put into your baby's eyebrow. A schedule would let you build in that five minutes you know Johnny always takes anyhow, and it may let you feed the cat before Johnny gets up.

Once you've conquered planning one meal, expand the schedule to the week, because if you look at the circle of "What's for breakfast?" it could be connected to its own schematic. Who's shopping, what's the budget, what are foods to eat? Making a schedule for the week allows you to plan meals, even meals you may have to eat in the car on the way to hockey practice.

Schedules save money too. If you make a schedule of meals, then make a list for the grocery store, you'll spend less and waste less than if you just show up at the grocery store hungry. The downside of schedules is that

[27] Stephen H. Kellert, *In the Wake of Chaos: Unpredictable Order in Dynamical Systems* (University of Chicago Press, 1993), 32.

making them is an investment of time. Sometime during the current business and chaos of life, you'll have to find 10 minutes to write out the plan for the week. Make sure to include activities along with meals. No point in roasting the chicken on Tuesday if you're going from soccer practice to gymnastics to Girl Scouts. A chicken dinner isn't going to work that day.

When I talk to parents about scheduling, they understand that writing out a schedule makes sense. But most don't do it. Most are stuck in the feeling of being overwhelmed, and maybe they've tried a schedule before that lasted until the ink was dry and then something happened (Fate) to make the schedule irrelevant. The road to hell is paved with schedules and to-do lists, right? Not necessarily. If making a schedule for a week seems impossible, just make a schedule of lunches for the week or just make a schedule for what lunches will be on Monday, Wednesday, and Friday. Don't try to be perfect. In fact, since we're in this for the long haul, it's okay to only plan meals for one day a week, and then as you get that feeling of power that it brings, expand it to another day and then another.

It may be worth sticking a Post-it note on this section, just to remind you to consider your locus of control as you make changes. Your family is going to the Island of Healthy Living. You're the one who's going to buy the tickets.

# ~ CHAPTER 9 ~

# Danger:
# Curves Ahead

Change is good. Change is hard. Change, change, it does a body good. The problem with change is, well, it's different – from what you did before, for the past year or the past decade; maybe it's even different from what you did your entire life. To lead your family to the Island of Healthy Living, though, some things will have to change.

As you make changes, you're going to encounter resistance about what you're trying to do. You're going to get push-back in all the areas: screen time, SSBs, activity, and what's on the plate. Depending on the support from the other adults around and depending on the personality of your children, you may get so much resistance that you'll feel like you're stuck in a trash compactor. At least temporarily, your children may dig in their feet to oppose any change, maybe by gorging on Twinkies now that they're back on sale, maybe by holding a sit-in Survivor episode marathon, and they'll say that there's no way in heckola they're moving to some stinking island if they have to eat their vegetables to do it. They'll stand there with their arms crossed and that pouty expression every parent loves to see, and they'll wait to see how serious you really are. All of that opposition will make you reconsider whether you really want anything to change. The thought will cross your mind that the Island of Healthy Living is likely similar to Atlantis, which sank anyhow and probably didn't exist in the first place. At some point, you'll want to say, "Forget it. It's impossible." Welcome to initiating change.

| **WHAT TO EXPECT TO HEAR AS YOU MAKE CHANGES:** |
| --- |
| **1.** I'm hungry. |
| **2.** It doesn't taste good. |
| **3.** It's too hard |
| **4.** Why do I have to do it and he doesn't? |
| **5.** It's too hard. (yes, this repetition is intentional.) |

Let's switch topics. Consider kids and guns. No matter which side you're on in the gun-control debate, you would never let your 3-year-old play with a loaded gun and say, "It's too hard to get up and take it away right now. I'll just let her play with it tonight and take it away tomorrow." You would do whatever you had to do to take the gun away. No matter what kind of tantrum your child threw when you removed her "toy," you would take it away because her life would be at stake. Now go back to obesity. Would you take away a bottle of juice even if your toddler cried for it?

I know you've already predicted where I'm going with this, but hear me out. Lots more people die from obesity-related diseases (diabetes, heart disease, stroke) than from firearm injuries.[28] In fact, in 2009, more than 25 times the number of people died from preventable chronic diseases than from firearms. Again, I'm not making an argument either way about guns and legislation, I'm simply pointing out that without making drastic changes to our lifestyles, we've got a good chance of ending up dying of a cause that is just as preventable as keeping a gun from a toddler. This is your child! Maybe we should feel the same sense of urgency about her health as we do about her safety.

## SLOW CHANGE

Since change is hard (oops, did I say hard? I meant character building), I want to remind you to not dive into all four areas of ADK 2015 at once, and I'll warn you again to NOT aim for perfection in any of the areas. The goal is NOT to be perfect, but just to be healthy. I'll also say again that the argument is not to lose weight (I'll try to mention that every few pages). That's been borne out by a few studies lately that say being slight-

28 Kenneth D. Kochanek, Jiaquan Xu, Sherry L. Murphy, Arialdi M. Miniño, Hsiang-Ching Kung, "Deaths: Final Data for 2009," National Vital Statistics Reports 60, no. 3 (2011):38-40.

ly overweight is healthier than thin. Since I'm not certain the researchers excluded methamphetamine addicts from the thin category, I don't know whether I buy into the results, BUT it does illustrate that if we shoot for certain numbers, we're going after a moving target and we're very likely to miss the big prize.

---

# THINK SMALL!

**Another reason to make small changes is because the effect can be exponential!**

**As one area is improved, it will impact the others. For instance, as screen time goes down, physical activity goes up!**

---

If you've ever gone on a diet yourself, think of how long the diets lasted that involved eating only lettuce, or only chicken. If you started the diet on Monday, by Wednesday you're sneaking out of bed at midnight and gorging on the candy corns you've stashed in the top of the pantry, which you justify since corn is a vegetable and lettuce is a vegetable, and A = C, so candy corns should have been part of your diet to start with. Ultimately, what we want is a healthy lifestyle, not an extreme way of living, and the good news is that even though change usually has to happen to get to a healthy lifestyle (hello island breeze, goodbye arctic jet stream), it's a kind of change that is sustainable and incremental.

---

**The changes you make for your family will only last when they become habits. That's why it takes so long to make changes stick, and why it's important to focus on one area at a time before you move on to the next.**

---

While writing this book, I decided that perhaps I should go ahead and lose the 10 extra pounds I've been carrying around my midsection since my last child was born. I figured I could tell people it was baby weight only for the first four years after my baby was born, but after that, I needed to call it something else. To lose the weight, I knew what I had to do: get rid of the box of candy in my office and limit my lunchtime portion sizes to something smaller than what a T. rex might consume in a week.

But I didn't chuck the box of candy in the trash can when I finally decided to change. I'm not that wasteful! Instead, I ate less and less chocolate every day until the box was empty, then I simply didn't refill it, although one day I will. Every time I felt that urge to open the candy box, which occurred every 15 minutes or so, I munched on a carrot stick instead. I did this around the holidays, which made my staff believe I had willpower of steel. About the same time, a longtime staff member was giving a new nurse a rundown of the office, and she referred to me by saying, "She won't eat chocolate; she's on a diet." I was not on a diet!! Instead, I was simply getting back to my healthy weight, but without dieting; I was just looking at the habits I'd acquired over the years, picked two that I knew weren't healthy, and decided to make a change. It wasn't a diet, it was a change in eating habits, and hopefully one I'll continue for years to come. I still ate chocolate! And I still made sticky buns for Christmas morning. Even small changes, like altering snacking habits, and cutting portion sizes at lunchtime, were difficult, though, and I'd never succeed long term even with 10 piddly pounds if I tried to make extreme changes.

I would expect that for this book to help point the way to the beautiful island you're hoping to get to, you're going to have to live with it for about a year. By the end of the year, it should be marked up, dog-eared, stained, and generally well-used. For a successful change toward a healthy lifestyle, the fastest someone can generally move is about one habit change per three months. A relatively small habit change, like decreasing portion size, may need to be maintained for even longer than three months, because you'll need to keep the change up until, well, until the new behavior becomes the habit and reverting back to your old ways becomes a change

---

# TAKE TIME TO CHANGE

Tackle small changes in two-week increments
before moving to another.

For bigger changes, give six to12 weeks before
adding something else.

Some examples: changing from whole milk to skim milk may take
six weeks to get used to, but changing from 2% to skim milk
should only take two weeks. Walking every day after supper may
take weeks to establish as a habit, but turning the TV off while
you eat could be easier.

---

Once health becomes a habit[29], you won't have to concentrate on specific areas anymore, but whatever change you made – let's say it was portion size – that habit can be maintained while you move onto altering something else. Habits can be ingrained into a family's way of living so they become automatic, and once they're automatic, there's no more push-back, no more opposition! It's a given that no matter what, most days Dr. Heidi will eat fresh fruits and veggies for a snack instead of candy, so everyone might as well quit asking.

Slow change is important for three different reasons. First, it's important for our psyches to be successful in the short term. No soda for a day? Wooohooo! Party! A short-term goal of no soda for a day is so much easier to attain than a goal of no soda for a year. But just as importantly, slow changes will also be sustained. Who wants to put effort into a healthy lifestyle if you're going to forget it after the first holiday season and you have to make the same New Year's resolution again this year? ("I'm eating ONLY lettuce on Mondays. This year, I'm really going to do it." Plus, on a much,

---

[29] A "habit," according to Dictionary.com, is an acquired behavior pattern regularly followed until it has become almost involuntary. For example, the habit of looking both ways before crossing the street.

much larger scale (think butterfly effect), you're creating changes for future generations. Yes, you want your child and your family to be healthy today, but you don't want your grandchildren to go through the machinations you had to go through to get there. (Remember that question in the last chapter about what are our goals for a society?) You want your grandchildren to be on autopilot! You want them to establish habits from birth that are healthy.

Finally, slow change is much less likely to get the knee-jerk reaction of "No way, not me!" and "Pass the 2-liter sugar-sweetened beverage. I'm never going to drink just water!"

---

# FIND A CHEERLEADER!

Who are the people willing to support and encourage you through thick and thin?

Those are the people who need to be around while you make changes! Those are the people to invite to dinner, share recipes with, talk to about struggles.

A cheerleader might be a mentor—someone who has been down the road before and come out successful on the other side. For instance, another parent whose children are older now, but when they were younger, they threw their vegetables across the kitchen table and refused to even look at broccoli.

---

## PRACTICAL WAYS TO MAKE CHANGES LAST

To make the changes last, do the following:

1. **Define goals.**
2. **Keep your motivation for change in mind.** (Write your dreams out, then post them on the fridge, tattoo them onto the hand that you use to reach into the potato chip bag, or set automatic text mes-

sages to send to yourself.)

**3. Find a cheerleader.**

**4. Have a "long-haul" mentality.**

**5. Get "buy-in."**

---

# RED FLAGS

The naysayers have to be given the boot for a while! Or at least they can't be invited to eat and exercise with you. Trouble is, naysayers can be cloaked in love and sometimes they're hard to recognize. Here are a few things they're going to say:

*"He's hungry, just give him what he'll eat."*

*"I fed you white bread and you turned out okay."*

*"It's important to have a treat and get rewarded."*

*"It's too cold to go outside."*

*"I don't like vegetables either!"*

*"No one wants to exercise in the rain."*

*"It's too expensive to eat healthy."*

*"This isn't going to work."*

---

Depending on your personality, and your innate parenting style, you'll tend to promote change by either dictating it or by acquiring "buy-in." My innate tendency is to create a dictatorship – not one in which I am on the receiving end of the laws. My preference is to be in charge. It's taken years of personal growth and a few bazillion self-help books to effect change in my parenting style and to alter my initial responses to people around me so that now I promote any change in my family by trying to get "buy-in."

That's a business term, the idea being that people who are financially invested in a business are much more likely to work hard and they'll be more dedicated to the success of the business. You want your family members to be invested in the success of a healthy lifestyle. You want them to help you pack for the trip to the island. You won't get change, at least not long- term, happy, unresentful change, by dictatorial tactics. You need "buy-in." And while it might be nice to go around and ask for a few hundred dollars from each family member, it isn't very realistic. You need to get something else: a "virtual buy-in" in the form of engagement to ensure their commitment.

Let me give an example of buy-in regarding nutrition, specifically for when you start working on the numbers 0 and 5 of ADK 2015. There are at least four areas in which you can engage your family and garner buy-in. You can ask for help in meal planning, food acquisition, meal preparation, and presentation. For instance:

- Who decides what's to eat for breakfast and dinner?
- Who goes to the grocery store?
- Who picks out the cantaloupe in the produce department?
- When it gets down to it, who's thumping the fruit to check for freshness?
- Who cooks?
- Who brings the food to the table or fixes the plates?

If the answer to all those questions is always the same person, then there's going to be very little buy-in when that same person tries to make changes in any aspect of family nutrition. But even a 3-year-old can enjoy a trip to the grocery store (God bless the marketers who turned grocery carts into racing cars), and a 5-year-old would love to use a salad spinner or stir a casserole. If you have a child who's even vaguely creative, she will light up if you ask her to arrange food on the plate so it's in an appealing presentation. And there's not much that makes kids smile at dinnertime faster than when they can give their mashed potatoes a smiley face made out of carrot sticks or their hamburger can be shaped in the initial of their first name. (Don't push back now! Don't say, "But she'll never eat the carrot sticks." All you're trying to do for the first step is to get engagement, not ingestion.)

---

**POSITIVE SELF-TALK**

Check out the pickthebrain.com blog for seven steps to positive self-talk:

**1. Eliminate internal negative chatter.**

**2. Positive affirmations.**

**3. Positive scripts.**

**4. Replace negative influences with positive ones.**

**5. Present-tense messages.**

**6. Confront fears.**

**7. Focus on enjoyable moments.**

---

If you're like me (all together now, say type A), you're going to have to accept the messiness that occurs when the kids get involved. There's potential for an orange avalanche in the produce department because every toddler knows the physics behind fruit stacking, and she knows which orange, once removed, will send the rest rolling to the floor. She's going to splatter tomato sauce on the floor when she stirs, and she's going to get the salad spinner going so fast that it will take off like a UFO and scatter arugula across the countertops. It's okay. It's okay. You're in this for the long haul.

On the other hand, if you're looking for engagement of family members in various realms of activity (the 2 and 1 of ADK 2015), it's worth asking what kind of activity they enjoy. If they like hiking, don't sign them up for a swimming course at the Y and browbeat them into attending. The long and short of it is, as you make changes, any kind of changes at all, you're going to face resistance, but that push-back can be minimized by making small changes over a long period of time and by getting engagement from your family in the form of participation or "buy-in."

# ~ CHAPTER 10 ~

# Beyond ADK 2015

ADK 2015 all started with me, another pediatrician, the director and community resource advocate for our community's local medical home pilot, and the director of the local Health Department. We brainstormed ways to impact obesity in our community and we dreamed big about what could happen. Now, once a month, representatives from our patient-centered medical home pilot (including administration, social workers, and nurses) meet with representatives from three pediatric practices, the director of the local fitness center, the director of a rehabilitation center, school representatives, dietitians, Health Department representatives and nutritionists, and we talk about childhood obesity in our community and our next steps.

I would never have envisioned the passion and the energy that could be created around this topic, and in 10 years our community will be significantly different because of it. We're already seeing changes in individual lives. But before we looked at our community, we had to look at our own families. We had to make changes in our own homes before we could impact others. Once we did, we simply had to expand our family, and that has an infinite number of possibilities. We need to challenge and set examples for our day cares and our churches and our schools. We have to support legislation that encourages activity and creates walkable cities, that makes choosing health easy instead of difficult. We need systems and co-ops that provide healthy foods at affordable prices. We need oases instead of food deserts. We need sustainable CSAs[30] to produce year-round food for communities.

We have to help each other. I'm a rotten bread maker. I know that. So does my friend who's using my latest loaf of bread for a doorstop. It's hard to implement changes, so instead of saying I'll never make bread, I need to reach out to a friend who is an exceptional bread maker and have him come teach me how to do it.

[30] Community Supported Agriculture involves agreements between consumers and farmers in the same area. Members of the CSA (the consumer) purchase shares in a local farmer's harvest. The arrangement provides local economic and agricultural benefits to the community as well as high quality local foods to the consumer.

After you master the principles of ADK 2015 in your own family, ask yourself, who else is in your community? Where can you teach the concepts of ADK 2015? Where can you learn the next steps? Who can you teach to bake bread? Does your town have a community garden? Do the kids in your child's school know what it's like to dig in the dirt?

ADK 2015 is a lifestyle change, and by now you know it works. In one year, with about three-month increments of relatively small changes, your family can return to being healthy; you can start living on that beautiful island. And once you're there, start bringing your friends. The nasty F word doesn't have to mean "forever" for anyone.

# ～ A P P E N D I X ～

# What We Talk About
# When We Talk About Obesity

## BMI AND THE BOOGEYMAN

The medical diagnosis associated with weight problems is *obesity*. It's an ugly name, but it isn't quite as bad as "fat." That said, when we talk about weight, some people shut down when they hear certain words. From my standpoint, the definitions are only the beginning of the conversation. We can call weight troubles whatever we want – with the caveat that soften-

{ *Doctors often talk about* **weight problems** *the way parents talk about* **the boogeyman.**

ing the blow is only important if it helps someone listen.

There's a whole list of euphemisms for fat, and although they're entertaining, they do what most euphemisms do: blunt the truth. It's a common response to life and death scenarios. The argument against euphemisms is that blunting the truth isn't beneficial when change is urgently needed. For example, a soldier wouldn't warn the new recruit about incoming missile attacks by saying, "Better get down, Frank, I believe there are some powder puffs coming our way." Instead, he'd scream something like "Incoming!"

Too often, though, doctors take the extreme opposite of euphemisms and talk about weight problems like parents talk about the boogeyman. The following may sound familiar:

"If he doesn't lose weight, he's going to die."

Or "You should only put him on a diet if you want him to live past 20."

Conversations starting like that are incredibly damaging to a patient's self-esteem, not to mention what they do to doctor-patient relationships.

Although being direct is sometimes helpful and necessary, being cruel never is, and lots of times, being direct is detrimental to motivating change.

> *"He's not fat, he's...*
> *Ample.*
> *Big-boned.*
> *Chunky.*
> *Fluffy.*
> *Healthy.*
> *Husky.*
> *Just like his cousin.*
> *Solid.*
> *Stocky.*
> *Thick. "*

Plus, conversations in the doctor's office regarding weight problems usually have less urgency than incoming missiles, and the boogeyman logic invalidates the doctor. If the child is 4 and looks just like his Uncle Teddy, who is 45, then the parent knows the threat isn't immediate. I mean, let's say your child is 8 years old. I'll bet he didn't go from the bottom of the growth curve to the top in one season. What kind of urgency is there in a process that has taken eight years? Most of the time, conversations about weight are semi-urgent.

If opening a conversation about weight by calling someone "solid" or by talking about joint pain instead of numbers, well, if that's what it takes to get a child healthier, I'm okay with that. And I'm also okay if it takes months or years of talking as long as we're moving in the right direction.

$$\text{BMI} = \frac{\text{Weight in Pounds}}{\text{Height in Inches}^2} \times 703$$

Weight categories are defined by something called BMI, body mass index. It's a number anyone can calculate by plugging height and weight measurements into a specific formula. The calculation is a translation of the idea that tall people should weigh more than short people. If you know your child's height and weight (or your own), you can identify your weight category based on BMI. Match the number up with a chart, and voila! You just discovered whether your family is vertically challenged or not!

## ADULT BMI

| Calculated BMI | Weight Category |
|---|---|
| < 18.5 | Underweight |
| 18.5 - 24.9 | Normal |
| 25 - 29.9 | Overweight |
| > 30 | Obese |

If a doctor talks to you about BMI, he or she will probably use a nasty O word as well — "obese," or its cousin, "overweight." Part of the reason we use those words is because the ICD codes (the codes your insurance company uses to assign payment to doctors) use them. The definitions of overweight and obese are determined by the BMI calculation[5].

[5] National Heart, Lung and Blood Institute, Obesity and Physical Activity Guidelines (1998), xiv.

For children, there is a wide range of what is considered a normal BMI, and that range is standardized on a percentile base, just like height, weight, and head circumference. So when your child's BMI is given, it will also be stated as a percentile. The idea is to compare our children with their peers, but parents shouldn't interpret the BMI and growth chart percentile ranking the same way as a school grading scale. In the case of BMI, 98% is not an A.

Percentiles are a comparison. If a child has a 50% BMI, about half of the kids his age and sex have a higher BMI and about half have a lower one. The 50% BMI doesn't mean he failed; it means he's in the middle. And being in the middle doesn't mean much until we compare it with how the child has grown over time.

| CHILDHOOD BMI | | |
|---|---|---|
| BMI% | Weight Category | Color Zone |
| < 5% | Underweight | Blue |
| 5% < 85% | Healthy weight | Green |
| 85% < 95% | Overweight | Yellow |
| ≥ 95% | Obese | Red |

The percentile is used instead of a set number (like for adults) because children grow! A BMI of 16 might be horribly excessive for a 4-year-old, but underweight for a teenager. Using percentiles normalizes BMIs. Percentiles between 5% and 85% are considered healthy. A BMI between 85% and 94% is defined as overweight, and greater than or equal to 95% is obese. Those are medical definitions, and trust me, I've handed out enough visit summaries to know that the diagnosis of "obese" can be just as upsetting to parents as the word "fat" is to kids.

In the end, I'd rather not use the word "obese," although for now, if I want to get paid, I'm stuck with it. But when I select the diagnosis as a billing code and send it off to the insurance company, the parents and children who read that diagnosis hear the word "fat." In the end, what matters is whether there is a health problem, not what a number is or what words we use to describe the number.

| BMI is read as a percentile in children, since children grow! |
|---|
| 6-year-old boy with BMI of 20 = Obese |
| 12-year-old boy with BMI of 20 = Healthy Weight |
| 8-year-old girl with BMI of 15 = Healthy Weight |
| 16-year-old girl with BMI of 15 = Underweight |

BMI is only one tool to help assess health. It's easy to measure and non-invasive, and a patient and doctor can follow the trend of the number, whether a child is crossing weight categories (for example, from healthy to overweight, or overweight to obese). But BMI doesn't always reflect the true health of a child, and the numbers need to be matched up with the clinical picture. There are serious problems with using BMI as the be-all end-all to determine a child's health status. BMI is simply a starting point, and a complete evaluation should include comprehensive physical fitness and nutrition assessments.

| Calculated BMI | "Old" Definition | "New" Definition |
|---|---|---|
| BMI 85% to < 95% | At risk of being overweight | Overweight |
| BMI> 95% | Overweight | Obese |

I can't tell you the number of times I've reviewed a BMI chart with a parent, and the number for the kid (a total potato-chip junkie who watches TV 15 hours a day) is sitting on the healthy weight line, about to tip over into the abyss of overweight, and the mom is doing a victory dance because she's been vindicated. Her child isn't fat! Sitting on the line isn't healthier than being just on the other side of it. The terms are arbitrary, and with the risk factors of that child's lifestyle, I don't care much whether he is in the "healthy weight zone" – he's got major work to do on his health. Someone, or some committee, had to decide which BMI numbers needed the label "obesity" and which range would be considered a "healthy weight." That means a line had to be drawn somewhere, and depending on which side of the line your child falls on, you may be doing the happy dance or crying and vowing you're only going to feed him organic carrot sticks for the rest of your life.

Not only are the terms associated with BMI arbitrary, but the definitions also change over time, and with the change in definition sometimes comes a change with names as well. What used to be "at risk for overweight" is now plain old "overweight." And when the term "obesity" was added to the definitions, a whole lot of people woke up one morning and found out they were fat![6] So if you think you know which category you're in, check back, because it could change overnight.

| **PROBLEMS WITH USING BMI:** |
| --- |
| It's arbitrary (so the definitions can change). |
| It's based on nineteenth-century Europeans. |
| It's skewed by muscle mass. |
| It doesn't consider the location of fat. |

BMI also doesn't take into account the composition of a body. An elevated BMI usually correlates to a high fat content, but muscular, athletic kids could have a high BMI but have very little adipose, or fat, tissue. Arnold Schwarzenegger in his weight-lifting years probably had a high BMI. But he wasn't obese. Parents often use this fact to argue that BMI

[6] In June 1988, the National Institutes of Health began using BMI to categorize healthy or unhealthy weights. Overnight, the range of weights considered healthy changed, and people went to bed one morning at a healthy weight and awakened the next day labeled "obese"!

is not legitimate as it relates to their child. But many times I hear the argument applied to pre-teens, who physically don't have the ability to build as much muscle as teenagers or adults. I can really think of only a handful of patients over the years who truly fit the Schwarzenegger BMI model, and I was even uncertain about those.

> **JOKE:** If someone's BMI is > 30, and he wants to improve his health, he can either *lose weight* or *grow taller.*

BMI is also based on nineteenth-century (Caucasian) Europeans, and it doesn't consider the location of the fat. Someone has much higher health risks if she has fat around her middle as opposed to in her thighs. If you're adamant that BMI doesn't accurately reflect your child's health, you might be right. But it could be dangerous to totally discredit one measurement. It is wiser to follow it along and see how it trends over time. Besides, muscular people can easily become fat if they stop exercising but keep eating the same number of calories.

In the ideal world, we wouldn't have to worry about imperfect calculations and would simply measure fat, actual fat, the kind that muddles up our middles and invades our thighs and rear ends and gives us spare tires and muffin tops. But that would involve water displacement, or air displacement, and no one wants to dip kids in a swimming pool every time they go to the doctor's office. Can you imagine assessing fat content by water displacement?

"Step onto the scale, Sam." He does.

"Stand against the wall, Sam. Heels down, all the way back." He gets his height measured.

"Okay, then... clothes off. Strip down, Sam, and into the pool you go!"

# A **healthy lifestyle** will look the same *no matter what* a healthy weight is defined as! }

Calipers and abdominal-circumference tools can also help assess fat and distribution of fat, but everything, even BMI, is a measurement that is only assumed to correlate with health. No measurement is perfect, and all the target ranges are based on populations, not individuals. When it comes down to just one person whose BMI is at issue, the measurement may not be perfect. But my new favorite saying is: *don't let perfect be the enemy of good.*

When we consider how discretionary BMI is, and when we think of how definitions can change overnight (or at least after the latest committee meeting), the tendency may be to throw up our hands and say it doesn't matter. In addition, if we consider a high BMI number "bad," it can be an easy jump for some people to consider those who are overweight "bad" as well. But the idea of correlating personal worth with appearance is terrible. Obesity has such a stigma associated with it that many of us can't look past someone's weight and see a brilliant artist or a cutting-edge scientist or, very simply, a beautiful soul. But I would argue that the problems with using BMI to measure obesity help emphasize a main point: we shouldn't focus on weight at all or we'll be aiming at a moving target.

We do need to acknowledge being overweight as a potential problem and a risk, and maybe even a part of a spiritual hunger we aren't satiating, but specific numbers and appearances shouldn't be our ultimate target. For better or worse, right now the calculation and the definition of BMI is what we have to work with when we're talking about weight. The Centers for Disease Control, and therefore doctors (because we're too busy seeing patients to haggle over formulas), use BMI to define overweight and obesity. If we consider the definitions with respect and some circumspection, they can be a starting point for a conversation about healthy living. To fix the problem of obesity, we'll need to focus on achieving a healthy lifestyle, which will look the same no matter what the Centers for Disease Control or the National Institutes of Health or any other healthcare agency defines as a healthy BMI!

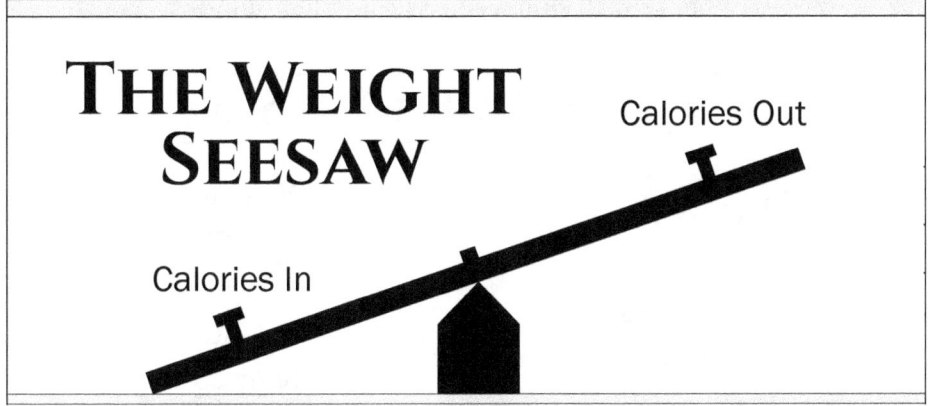

After we point a finger at BMI, put it in its place of useful but not perfect, and start tracking it as relates to our children's health, we must also look at the components of what lifestyle helps a child achieve and maintain a healthy weight. The truth is that weight is like a seesaw. Calories that a person eats are on one side, and calories that the person uses are on the other side. When the two sides even out, weight is stable. The problem is, the application is not that simple. In fact, I've pretty much given up on the seesaw example for anything other than the basic beginning conversation about how weight gain happens. One problem with the seesaw is that it naturally goes back and forth, specifically during the toddler years of grazing and during rapid times of growth when kids pack in the calories right before they shoot up in height. It can be difficult for a parent to distinguish a "spurt" from a harmful eating pattern. If I look at my own kids, the youngest one is always in the pantry saying she's hungry, and the older one seems to use food as a means to an end. The latter will eat if it's going to give her energy and keep her alive, but otherwise she can do without it. When my older daughter, the "means-to-an-end" child, says she's hungry, I'm going to believe it. With the one that's always in the pantry to start with? Well, I'm usually saying things like "Come play a game first" or "Wait a little bit and see how you feel." (She's usually really hungry for the first few days of her growth spurts since I think her hunger is habit).

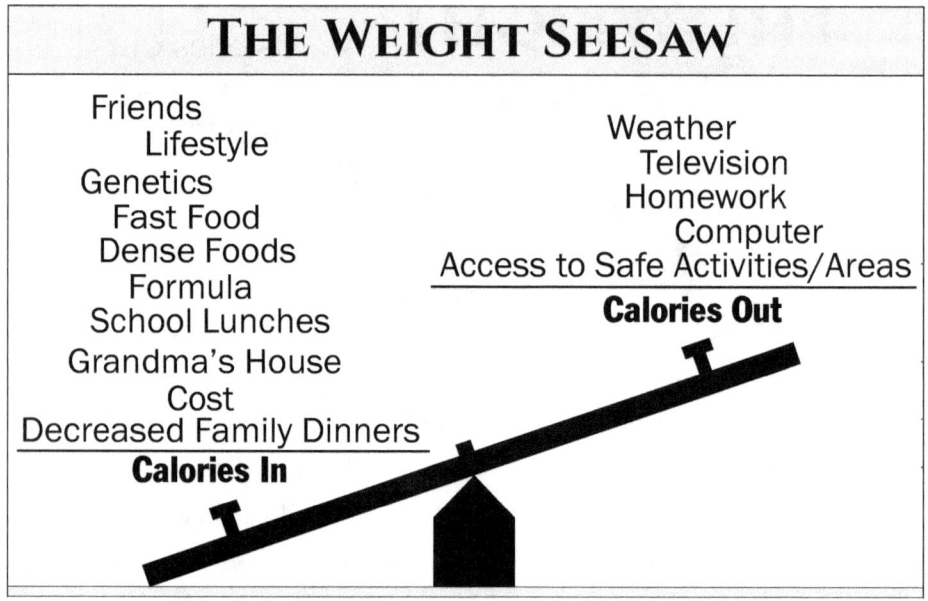

THE WEIGHT SEESAW

Friends
Lifestyle
Genetics
Fast Food
Dense Foods
Formula
School Lunches
Grandma's House
Cost
Decreased Family Dinners
**Calories In**

Weather
Television
Homework
Computer
Access to Safe Activities/Areas
**Calories Out**

It's also challenging to fight against external factors that unbalance the seesaw. Take "calories out," for instance. We live in the North Country of upstate New York, so six months of winter discourages us from getting outside and burning calories. If you live in Mississippi, though, six months of summer might be just as much of a barrier. And on the other hand, some kids may simply not have a safe place to play outside. Environment and limited opportunities to be active push the "calories out" end of the seesaw up or down depending on the issue. The other end of the seesaw, the "calories in" side, can be affected by environment as well; just think about how a fixed income or school lunches or snack time at the babysitter's may get in the way of equilibrium.

This is not the time to toss the book into a bowl of potato chips, throw up your hands, and climb up the pantry shelves to the bag of candy corns waiting to console you. Instead, as with BMI, you should use the good parts of the seesaw analogy and consider the different influences pushing the sides up and down as ways to identify problems and illuminate areas where you're going to get solutions!

For instance, are six months of winter keeping your family from exercising? It could be a great opportunity to push outside your own comfort zone and learn about snowshoeing or create an entertaining indoor exercise plan. No safe location for outdoor play in your neighborhood? Maybe it's time to travel a few extra subway stops to get to a different park or find an organization or parent group with like-minded concerns and brainstorm together.[7]

## FAMILY METABOLISM

While doctors tend to talk about the boogeyman and all the bad things that will happen to kids who are in the red zone weight category, parents tend to talk about family. That is, they say that their child is "built like" someone else. Maybe it's mom, dad, or cousin Arnie. But essentially, what

{ **Metabolism** can be a *tool to help* us reach a *healthy weight.*

---

[7] Mothers on the Move, for instance, is a grass-roots effort in the Bronx, focused on finding safe places for children to play in the city, where there is only one acre of green space per 1,000 people.

I hear parents say is that their child's family just doesn't use food the way other people use food. Instead, those families savor every single unit of energy, even holding onto those units for an extended time and storing them up in the form of adipose tissue (a.k.a. fat). They aren't like their neighbors who only eat Twinkies and pasta and yet still look like fence posts. According to some parents, the whole family has a problem with metabolism, and really, we all just might as well accept the inevitable.

| HOW TO INCREASE METABOLISM |
| --- |
| Build muscle mass. |
| Have short, intense workouts. |
| Drink lots of water. |
| Eat small meals often. |
| Increase lean protein intake. |

Metabolism is a process that transforms food into energy. It consists of all the chemical reactions behind how we take food – a bowl of cereal or a steak, for instance – and convert it into the fuel our body needs for a walk around the block or a bicycle ride. The chemical reaction is constantly in flux for each person, and it varies based on age, gender, and what percentage of a person's body jiggles like a bowl full of Jell-O versus lean muscle mass. A fast metabolism is the holy grail of a healthy weight. Think of all the sales pitches for dietary supplements that promise to "Boost your metabolism!"

On my cynical days, I consider the explanation of a low metabolism as nothing more than an easy excuse for making poor lifestyle choices. It's a fantasy about why the pounds don't come off quite as easily for one person as for the next. After all, the kid in the family with the "slow" metabolism usually seems to be the one knocking back a few extra Oreos for a bedtime snack. But on my realistic days (and usually the few days I step on a scale to weigh myself), I think the metabolism argument is probably why losing post-pregnancy weight when I was 27 years old was a heck of a lot easier than when I was 37.

| WHAT AFFECTS METABOLISM |
| --- |
| Gender |
| Age |
| Size |
| Muscle Content |

In fact we can do simple things to get our bodies burning more calories, and our kids can do them as well. Some of the changes involve shifting diet (more fruits and veggies, more lean protein), and some involve changes in exercise routine (morning activity, anyone?). The important part is that metabolism is malleable, and it's going to be simultaneously a tool we can use and an obstacle along the way to a normal weight.

I'm not offering a set of Ginsu steak knives or a nifty extra gadget like a pickle picker for free if you order in the next 15 minutes, but you still can boost your child's metabolism, and it's something worth trying to change. Does that mean metabolism also affects how your child gains weight? Absolutely. But we don't have to focus on metabolism. If we focus all of our energy on creating a healthy lifestyle, we will ultimately change our metabolism for the better. Just like BMI, metabolism is worth considering, but we shouldn't make it our ultimate goal. It's going to be the end result anyhow.

## LAB TESTS

When you start the conversation with a doctor about your child's weight, chances are he'll recommend some lab tests. The Academy of Pediatrics recommends screening labs for all children at least once in their childhood, and those standard labs should include a cholesterol screening. So even if your child isn't struggling with his weight, he still needs his cholesterol level checked at least once before he heads off to adulthood. Cholesterol checks help screen for heart disease, and all children, even those without weight problems, need it drawn at least once. But if your child is overweight, he also needs to be checked for diabetes. It's one of the most common complications of weight problems.

| TESTS IF THE BMI > 85%<br>**Yellow or Red Zone** |
| --- |
| Blood pressure |
| Lipid profile<br>  - *Total cholesterol*<br>  - *HDL cholesterol*<br>  - *LDL cholesterol*<br>  - *Triglycerides* |
| Fasting glucose |
| Hemoglobin A1C. |

Diabetes is a disease created when the body can't make enough insulin to keep up with the load of sugar or carbohydrates coming in, or the body makes plenty of insulin (the part of the body that makes insulin is called the pancreas), but the cells that are supposed to respond to insulin ignore it because they've become resistant or immune. The latter is what used to be called type 2 diabetes, or adult-onset diabetes. Unfortunately, it is now very much applicable to children, and it is sort of like a teenager who has stopped hearing his parents tell him to clean his room. The message is getting sent, the cells have just stopped responding. Often, children who have weight problems also show signs of insulin resistance, the first step to becoming diabetic[8], and many are flat-out diabetic. Testing for diabetes may include checking fasting glucose levels and hemoglobin A1C (the percentage of hemoglobin in the blood that has glucose attached).

---

[8] Juvenile diabetes, which is often called type 1, is not caused by excess weight and dietary choices, but by an immune system attack on the pancreas.

Other levels to consider checking are thyroid hormone levels, specifically a thyroid screening hormone, and a free thyroxine. The thyroid gland is located in the front part of the neck, somewhere near the Adam's apple, and the gland has a lot to do with metabolism. If someone has hypothyroidism, she may gain weight even if she doesn't eat much. The pivot point on the seesaw is reset, so to speak, so very few calories "in" have to be followed by a disproportionate amount of calories "out" to maintain a balance.

## PARTS OF THE WHOLE

The pancreas is only one area of the body affected by an unhealthy lifestyle and too much weight. Actually, every organ system is affected by obesity! One of the kindest mentors I had in medicine spent a few minutes talking to me after we saw a very overweight woman. He pointed out how difficult it must be for the woman to do anything during the day – bathe, walk, or drive, for instance. And as physically difficult as it must have been, she had to do everything while many other people looked at her and treated her with a level of disgust that she didn't deserve.

It's no wonder that kids who weigh too much feel bad. Their bones ache; their muscles ache. Sometimes they can't breathe well, and their self-esteem is rock bottom. Their hearts hurt – figuratively and sometimes literally too.

Childhood obesity is the hot topic for the country right now, and in another year there will be a million more studies and research projects about it. Well, maybe not a million. But still. The studies are driving me crazy. A month ago, I switched my exercise routine to incorporate weights because one study said it would burn more calories, and since I do like an eggnog latte a few times a week around Christmastime, I thought a shortcut to calorie burning was in order. A week later, a study said that burning fat is better done with aerobic exercise. Since I still want my lattes, I'm thinking I'm going to have to strap weights on all my extremities and get back on the treadmill. I dread the day a study comes out and says swimming is the best way to burn calories. If I keep following the studies and basing my exercise plan on what they say, I'm going to be running on a treadmill at the bottom of the pool somewhere.

Here's what I say. Forget about the studies. It's like chasing your tail if you're a Jack Russell terrier. Pretty useless. I'll save you time and personally guarantee (although not for $19.95 and a free asparagus peeler) that, in one way or another, the bazillion studies coming out next year are going to say the following:

1. Obesity is personally devastating.
2. Obesity costs families and society a ton of money.

Even though I've just destroyed all the grant applications out there for five hundred and one biochemists, it's worth pointing out that we already know the problem. We're about to walk through the ways to fix it.

## PARTS OF THE BODY AFFECTED BY OBESITY

| Organ System | Disease |
| --- | --- |
| Endocrine | Diabetes<br>Hormone Imbalances<br>  (Hyperandrogenism) |
| Genitourinary | Early Puberty<br>Irregular Menstruation |
| Cardiac | High Blood Pressure<br>Stroke<br>Coronary Artery Disease<br>Enlarged Heart |
| Gastrointestinal | Non-alcoholic Fatty Liver<br>Gallstones<br>Reflux |
| Respiratory | Sleep Apnea<br>Pneumonia |
| Orthopedic | Blount's Disease<br>Slipped Capital Femoral Epiphysis |
| Dermatologic | Skin Abscesses |
| Psychiatric | Depression |

# About the author

Dr. Moore lives on a farm in upstate New York in the foothills of the Adirondacks.

She connects with readers by email and can be reached for speaking engagements at hjmoore394@gmail.com

Her website is heidimooremd.com

www.ingramcontent.com/pod-product-compliance
Lightning Source LLC
Chambersburg PA
CBHW071716170526
45165CB00005B/2039